90 Days of Heat

Freedom Through Moksha

90 Days of Heat

Freedom Through Moksha

David Matthew Brown

BOOKS

Winchester, UK
Washington, USA

First published by O-Books, 2015
O-Books is an imprint of John Hunt Publishing Ltd., Laurel House, Station Approach,
Alresford, Hants, SO24 9JH, UK
office1@jhpbooks.net
www.johnhuntpublishing.com

For distributor details and how to order please visit the 'Ordering' section on our website.

Text copyright: David Matthew Brown 2014

ISBN: 978 1 78279 785 2

A CIP catalogue record for this book is available from the British Library.

Design: Lee Nash

Printed in the USA by Edwards Brothers Malloy

We operate a distinctive and ethical publishing philosophy in all
areas of our business, from our global network of authors to
production and worldwide distribution.

CONTENTS

Foreword

A man, an ex-husband, a father, a son, and a naked mystic. These are a few of the things I learned of a man sitting on a bench at the yoga studio one day. This man was David Matthew Brown and he was clearly in a place of being open to a journey and wanted to share his experiences along the way. We initially discussed the idea of completing 30 straight days of hot yoga. He explained that he planned to document and blog each day going forward. What may have started as a comfortable way of merging into a new life experience became a collection of honest feelings, raw emotions, pivotal breakthroughs and human moments. David's desire to share each day through his blog, the naked mystic, initially had us all a bit concerned as we explained to David that he could not take the hot yoga classes in the nude.

Fortunately, David arrived on his mat day after day after day fully clothed. I have seen many people gift themselves the idea of a consistent practice and life simply gets in the way. Work, school, relationships, the unknown emergency, insecurity, vulnerability, change, and other life events are all things that can shift our energy and focus from our practice. While these things were all present in David's journey you are about to learn how dedication and a deep willingness to understand our bodies and breath can take us further than our minds could ever imagine. Breath by breath David's practice develops into a true inspiring account of life and reality, becoming a testament to the evolution of a human being one breath, one movement, and one day at a time. On the mat, David explores many concepts and practices with an open and honest mind gaining insight and perspective along the way.

The writings, stories, and honest first-hand accounts of sweat and courage shared by David became a powerful tool, part of the greater process that is breath and the evolution and transformation of a human being. At one point I recall asking David where the reflection takes place to create the writings. I challenged him to allow the practice to be guided by the breath and to be present in the moment of sensation, as if we are fully consumed in practice with the intent to create something we may in fact be limiting ourselves of the possibilities to open, release, and receive. I challenged David to allow the experiences to set naturally and the documentation of the experiences or reflection process to take place elsewhere. In sharing, I learned in many cases that David would reflect during his walks to and from the studio. From the tears running down his face to encounters and signs from others, real life stuff interpreted in a positive light is what we are gaining in perspective here. It has been an incredible experience in getting to know David inside and outside of the hot room and look forward to the seeing what comes next from the naked mystic.

Joe Komar
Modo Yoga LA Instructor

The Jump

November 26th, 2010, and I had recently been separated from my wife and received a call from my Uncle Paul. "Hey, David, it's your uncle, congratulations you won a prize, give me a call, okay, bye."

My uncle has a wonderful sense of humor, so I called him back, and he explained that he, my aunt, and cousins were going skydiving the day after Thanksgiving and they would like me to go, though my aunt was having second thoughts.

I had never thought in my wildest dreams that first I would be going through a divorce, and second jumping out of an airplane, so I said, "Yes." What else could happen? So my almost three-year-old daughter and I drove down to a small airport by San Diego. As we arrived my daughter saw all the little planes, and asked what we were doing there, and I responded, "Well, Harper, your dad is going to jump out of plane?"

"Who's going to watch me?" she asked.

I smiled. "My aunt will watch you."

My uncle and aunt arrived, I was chosen to go first, and my heart was pounding, and my mind was dancing in fear. *What am I doing? This is nuts.* I would be jumping tandem. The man I was jumping with must have reassured me one hundred times, "David, I have made thousands of jumps, and this will be fun."

They strapped me up, and I came out and saw my daughter. We hugged tight, and she said, "Dad, I love you."

The man came out of the office in his gear. "David, lets go." I remember thinking they move fast, probably, and telling myself, *so you don't chicken out.* My aunt explained that Harper and the family would meet me at the final landing place. My daughter hugged me again and I watched them walk away.

Turning I went to talk to the man I would be jumping with. He again explained how many times he had jumped and then

I

took out his video recorder and pointed it at me. "David, how are you feeling about jumping?"

I responded quickly, "Good, I feel good," and stuck my tongue out to the camera.

The plane was tiny. On board would be a pilot, myself, the man I would be strapped to, and another man and jumper; five of us traveling in a tuna can, puttering up two miles high. The higher we flew, the more my mind started to race, and finally we arrived, hovering above the Pacific Ocean.

It was beautiful up there and I watched the other jumper sit on the edge of the plane, and then go. And after they jumped I heard, "Okay, David, we have to jump now, let's go." So we moved to the edge of plane, and I sat with my feet dangling over the edge. I heard directions being spoken to me, my mind screaming now, and like that, we jumped. All was quiet in me as we moved through the air, and I opened my eyes and looked out over the vast sky and down at the wonderful greens and browns of the fall season below me.

I signaled thumbs up to the camera that was on me, and said, "Wow," about fifty times. No words can describe the feeling of being up there.

The parachute shot open and we glided over Southern California, and as we were coming to land, I saw running beneath me my beautiful daughter Harper, yelling, "My dad can fly, my dad can fly."

As I landed, she came and jumped into my arms, and explained to me how she could see me flying in the air. The man asked if I would do it again, and I said, "Yes!"

We all decided to go for Mexican food. Harper and I jumped into my car and followed behind my uncle. Out of the blue, our car just gave up. Smoke billowed from the hood. My daughter asked me, "Dad, why is the car on fire?"

I said, "I have no idea." So we pulled off onto the shoulder.

Pulling up too, my uncle walked over, poked his head in, and said, "I'll tow it, and you guys can get in my car."

We hopped in my uncle's car. As we drove back to their house I remember thinking about my separation, moving out of the house, jumping out of plane, and then the thought came, *Now this*.

At that moment, it felt as if life kept giving me lemons. Over the next few months I would be mugged, become a caregiver, and endure family members that couldn't keep themselves out of the mediation between my wife and me. My Facebook became a posting ground of nonsense, from people who had no idea or sensitivity to divorce.

When two people decide to move on, it is quite difficult for both of them, whether they acknowledge it or not. A divorce is really a death. So many people are affected by it, not just the two people divorcing. In our case we had our daughter, who had grandparents, and then there were friends and family. Everyone believes they know what went on because they hear from one side, and so the process becomes bigger, personal, and in some cases ridiculous.

The divorce felt like the wind being knocked out of me, it really hurt, was painful, and I began to turn away from the world. I wanted to stay inside. I worked many jobs, and did the best I could to keep a positive outlook at work. It was difficult.

In particular, with divorce you feel raw inside. In fact so raw that you feel touchy, and so in front of my daughter, I kept up a strong sense of pride, trying to keep it together. And when she went to sleep, I had moments of where I just wept thinking about her living with two parents separately, and how hard that would be for her.

Early on in this period, I worked as a caregiver. I remember at the end of one long day at work, before I left, I had to change someone's diapers. The experience was very humbling. I came home to a Facebook message on my wall, from a family member, "David can't feed his daughter," which was not true. I remember reading that and crying. I was over the nonsense, over my thinking, over divorce, over people getting involved, over this life, and frankly just over it!

During the next three years, life offered me many ups and downs. As they came I dealt with them. But I had this overwhelming sense of shame, resentment, and guilt about my situation. How quickly my mind fed me stories of what happened, and every time the stories came, a part of me would bite like a fish, and in a flash my good day would become bad. I would re-live the situations in my mind.

After many meetings, therapy sessions, energy sessions, massages, and seeing my life from all different vantage points, I came across *Radical Forgiveness* by Colin Tipping. It was here that I started to feel a sense of relief. After I did his worksheet I noticed a weight being lifted. Finally after three years of resentment, there was actual movement happening. Actual forgiveness.

As I look back on that moment, I really feel as though the reason this actually started to work was I was ready, sincerely ready, to forgive. So I forgave it all. And as I forgave it, I began to have revelations and wisdom about why my life was unfolding the way it was and indeed had.

It felt great to have the burden off me.

I remember getting in my car to run errands around Los Angeles, and I felt as though I was renewed. I thought what could I do to mark this new beginning. As the thought appeared, I looked to my right and saw the sign, "Moksha Yoga," which was hot yoga. I thought to myself, *now that's interesting, I haven't done yoga for three years*. So I sat with the idea, but the idea didn't want to sit, it wanted to move, take action. As I had just started writing a blog, I thought it would be fun to do thirty straight days of hot yoga and blog on my experience every day. I would blog about my insights, struggles, and inspiration on the mat and how it was affecting me off the mat. I contacted Emily at the studio to let her know what I was doing; she loved the idea. So when I received her email that everything was good, I went and bought my unlimited month of yoga and started the next day.

After I went through forgiveness, there was, and still is, a tremendous sense of vulnerability. I used to believe vulnerability was weakness, but not anymore. Vulnerability is strength. By writing every day about my journey on the mat, I stayed open – stayed in the state of vulnerability – because what I learned on this 90 days of hot yoga is that life is not about holding on to anything, it flows no matter what. We are here to accept it, and then take action from the place of acceptance. I spent most of my life on this planet resisting, then proving others wrong, and then searching for approval: an unhealthy approach that worked for many years, but finally failed.

I invite you now into the 90-day journey, which originally started as 30 straight days and then moved to 90 straight days of hot yoga. Take your time with it. Use my journey to contemplate yours. We, meaning each of us, are in this together. Some days I offer little reminders, tools, on what I did to remain present. But each day offers one simple reminder – breath. Simple, but we take our breath for granted. Enjoy the journey. The journey I took over 90 days to arrive to where I have always been, but resisted.

I started this book explaining my skydiving experience, looking back that experience taught me that yes, I had fear in my mind, I was scared to jump, but I did. So you may be in a place right now where everything is going in the opposite direction to where you would like it to go. Take breath, and accept it. Accept where you are now. Accept the feelings, thoughts, and sensations that are happing inside you and be one with them. They are your real teachers. Witness them. Because if they are happening inside you, own it, they are your feelings. You matter, so your feelings matter.

Take your time with this journey. Remember you are already here, so be here fully, breathe, and enjoy!

90 Days Begin

Struggles, Inspiration, and Breathing

Day 1

Moksha and I

Today as I walked down to Moksha Yoga, there was an overcast sky, a nice breeze, and my thoughts. As I continued to walk to my first class, I felt I should set an intention: I would focus on my breath, and no matter what happened, I would rest in the breath.

I had found yoga in 1999 after I went to the doctor. The doctor explained I had high blood pressure and a couple of other things as well. He wanted to put me on drugs. I understood his intention, but there was no way was I going to take drugs. I thought there had to be another way. But I didn't have another way, so I let the doctor know that I would be back in six months, and if when I came back nothing changed, I would consider drugs.

A week later I decided to enter a yoga studio, change my diet, and I added to them Runyon Canyon for hiking. After two months of unlimited yoga, diet change, and hiking, I noticed a vast difference in my health and most importantly my mind. I went to the doctor, and guess what? Everything was normal. The doctor was shocked, he asked what I had done, I said I had cut out all red meat and fast food, added more fruit and vegetables, hiked, and incorporated yoga and meditation as well. From then on my diet changed to a vegetarian diet, hiking, yoga, meditation, and prayer work.

During my divorce, my diet changed, my body was craving meat again. I removed yoga because it seemed my body craved more physical work such as running and hiking, though I still meditated.

A couple of months later I did some forgiveness work, all the cravings stopped. No more running, some hiking, but what was amazing was this sense of now. Living and breathing. It was here that I started hearing my breath, contemplating my breath, allowing the breath, and no longer identifying with my mind. And when I did get caught up in my mind I would go to the breath, and so now my life is about "hearing the breath." When I hear my breath – really hear it – it reminds me of the ocean tide, it is beautiful.

I bring this up because in my first day of class today at Moksha, Joe our teacher brought up the importance of community and breathing; to me community is to commune with. In my practice today I spent time communing with my breath. Now don't misunderstand me, my practice was wobbly, tight, with only a couple of moments of fully expressing through my heart. But the breath was carrying me through each pose, no matter what. How I respond on my mat is how I respond in my life.

During my practice today a phrase kept creeping in, "God is closer than your breath," and what occurred to me was that the breath is who I am, or "breath I am." A couple of times I caught my self-reflecting from the vantage point of the breath; breath means *spiritus* in Latin, it is where we get the word *inspiration*, or *in breath*. As we breathe in life, and let it go, the inhale is "let" and the exhale is "go." The breath naturally moves with the flow of life without holding on. So by contemplating my breath in the practice, I was able to live in the body, and allow.

Joe our teacher mentioned freedom several times and our choice in it. I like that. I like that I have a choice in freedom, and that I can wrestle with myself on my mat in safety. Well on to day two…

Day 2

Getting My Sweat On!

It is day two of my 30 straight days at Moksha, and today's practice was filled with music. I continued to play with my breath, allowing the breath to guide me in the poses. Moksha is hot yoga, so you bring a towel, your mat, and water. The temperature of the room can rise to 102 degrees. At one point in the practice we were working on hips, my mind very active, and I suddenly became aware that I was gripping my towel like a baby holding a blanket. I smiled. The power of the breath is wonderful it really helps me to calm the mind when it starts to grip. I thought I might be a little tight from yesterday's practice but I actually felt good.

Everyday offers me new challenges, and today the challenge on my mat was breathing through my comfort zone and going into those places that were screaming. My comfort zone stops where the loud noises are. Meaning I prefer not go deeper. As I continued to breathe into and with and through those places I had a wonderful insight, "You're safe, nothing is going to hurt you here. You're on your mat," and I allowed myself to go inside, go inside to the sticky parts of me. Why not? We only live once so I might as well enjoy the opportunities as they arise.

I read a blog by a wonderful teacher and mystic Matthew Fox who said that in a capitalist land we are taught to be misers. To horde, to save up until we die then give it away. Then he suggested that love is a celebration that is always giving. Our job as lovers of love is to always be giving. I bring this up in regards to my practice: the more I give to it, the better I am. So when my thoughts are screaming, "YOU ARE NOT SAFE PULL BACK! AHHHHH!" I listen and keep breathing with it, and the noise subsides.

This is a wonderful acknowledgment for me. Most of the time I would run from these places, and now I am welcoming them in. Now you might not see the accomplishment, but I see it; and the more I continue to see me and hear me, the more I will stop demanding it from others and the world. Namaste...

Day 3

"No Breath, No Yoga"

Day three of my 30 straight days of hot yoga at Moksha in Los Angeles, California on La Brea and today I started on my mat with wonderful strength, and inner power formed and maintained with my breath. The breath works to ignite, enliven, and move the body. I love that we are encouraged to breathe and let the breath take us deeper. Our teacher today, Joe, played some cool tunes and mentioned, "No breath, no yoga." That really helped to inform me again of the power of the breath in my practice.

The breath for me is the connector between heaven and earth. It is about the whole being, incorporating the whole being into your practice. Sometimes yoga is looked at as just about the body, and the heaven aspect is left out. We need both heaven and earth in our practice to balance ourselves, especially in our lives filled with so many earthly things. Without heaven we become unbalanced in the world. Our breath, as Joe the teacher mentioned, is the "equalizer in our practice" and the bridge.

I am beginning to understand in my practice that by letting the breath into the parts of the body that may be tight, and resisting, I am letting in love. My breath accepts all life as it is. So for me the breath accepts the parts in me that are scared, hurt, shameful, or even guilty, and allows me to feel those places and release them. Especially in my hips, to breathe deep into them and allow the energy to move, it also seems to shake up lots of cellular memories too.

I have been noticing, too, that some old memories and feelings emerge. When I meditate on this, I receive guidance that it is just that, old memories that are looking to find their way out of the body.

In hot yoga I am recovering quickly each day and the body feels great and alive. Oh, thank you for the emails from both men and women who wanted to do naked yoga with me; sorry for the misunderstanding, I am doing hot yoga, with clothes on. Very flattered and it put a smile on my face. Well off to play with my daughter and see you tomorrow.

Day 4

Discover the Pose

Today I continued on to day four of 30 straight days of hot yoga. Before practice started, I lay down on my mat and closed my eyes. The room was quiet and I focused my attention on my breath coming into my nostrils and out. As I did this, an idea floated into my mind, "Discover the pose today." Then I thought, "Discover life."

How many times am I planning ahead? How many times am I dwelling on yesterday? How many times do I find myself in my head? Yet when do I give myself permission to discover life, or for that matter discover the pose, I feel more present.

Every pose in my practice is a discovery, with the breath guiding me to discover and accept each one as it is today. Christians have this same practice but they use the Our Father to practice with, reminding them that life is happening here and it is to be discovered as it is.

So today I used this idea to discover the intimate nature of the pose – allowing the breath to fully engage them. How quickly pride gets in and knocks you over. I found pride coming in and then I was knocked down. When the breath is fully engaged, I feel humbled in the pose, and the pose is discovered as it is.

This is important for me to discover how many times I expect people and situations to be different, and wanting them to change. It is up to me to accept life as it is, and I notice when I do that, my action steps are simple. But if I meet life and resist it, well life becomes a struggle. This happened in my practice today, on a back bend, the body was resisting and so I used my breath to allow the resistance to happen, why fight it. Funny, I noticed my shoulders blades come together and chest come out, and it felt like everything came from the inside out. Resisting is giving us an opportunity to rest. Resting in resisting is how we stretch ourselves.

Yoga offers us the invitation to discover the pose, and life offers us the same invitation – to discover life without war, defense, without the past. Life invites us to discover it as it is – staying open to discover the possibility that this is enough and so are you. If the pose is challenging me, rather than fighting and arguing with it, I discover it, meet it, and allow it to teach me: this seems to bring compassion to myself. Do I still fight it? Oh yes, but now I know when I am fighting, to stop, and breathe into the fight.

Day 5

"Stillness is Law"

As I went into day five of 30 straight days of hot yoga, I walked into my practice with a busy plate. I arrived early to collect myself, and in the process talked to some wonderful people who were waiting to take the class as well. I placed down my mat and then I lay on it and closed my eyes. I followed the flow of my breath and was amazed by the ordinariness of it, which led me to honor my mat more. Lying there before class, the reason occurred to me of why I love my mat so much. Once I get on it, I lose all identity to the world. On my mat I can just be. I am not a speaker, writer, author, blogger, single dad, student, or teacher; all of that drops away and I can just be ordinary.

Everything in my practice is calling me inward on my mat, every pose is inviting me to just be ordinary and release the need to be extraordinary. In a world where everyone is thriving to be extraordinary all the time, for an hour I can be ordinary. Yes there are moments in life and in the practice where we are called to be extraordinary, but those moments are few and far between. How exhausting to be extraordinary all the time. Constantly in a state of doing, needing approval, and proving to people all day long, that they are enough. I have discovered my moments come when I have the opportunity to speak in front of a group, but when I am done speaking, well, I go back to the ordinary. There is a famous Zen line, "Do laundry, carry wood, after enlightenment do laundry, carry wood." Ordinariness is an invitation to be okay now. We all would like to be just okay.

As the practice started the teacher asked us to breathe in the stillness, and at one point stated, "Stillness is law." I wish stillness were law. So I used the practice today to discover the stillness within it. I found many moments of stillness; I also found stillness towards the end of my practice. I had a chance to push through and decided to rest in the stillness of the breath and the sweat, and allow this to be as it is. I uncovered such gentleness with myself. I discovered an appreciation for who I am. I appreciated that I chose to stop and listen to myself, and not push, not will, not drive, which is a wonderful way to say, "I love you" to myself.

I am finding many lessons in my life lately, and the old ways I used to go about being in life are falling away. I am being called to spread my wings and leave the past at last where it belongs in the rear view mirror. I honor all that happened, and I am learning that forgiveness doesn't happen overnight, and that it is a process, and life gives you ample time to heal and then it invites you back into the fray. As I move into day six, I am honoring this journey of 30 days straight of hot yoga and admiring that no matter what happens I am showing up, and showing up fully. I honor you that read this.

Day 6

"Savor Now"

Approaching day six of 30 straight days of hot yoga at Moksha LA, I entered a long class. The teacher was wonderful. She set the intention early on to take it slow, to give ourselves these 90 minutes and "savor now." We started and really focused our attention on the pose, diving into it slowly, and with detail – savoring right now. At one point she announced, as we held a pose, "If you fall over, who cares." That made me chuckle. My mind raced quickly to all the times I have fallen over, and frankly nobody cares but us. My mind raced to the end of my marriage, which I felt was a huge fall, to starting over, to life not moving as I would like it, and wondering when it would actually move, to wondering if I would meet someone, blah blah, right? Because all these thoughts have a little bit of fact or truth that don't stand up to "now."

Every day for six days I have shown up on my mat, and have met the same 40 poses over and over, and in my meeting them, I have realized that each day brings new opportunities to rest a little deeper, relax into the chaos a little longer, and breathe. But most importantly allow my breath to move my practice.

Within my practice I am invited to leave my stories behind, leave yesterday, not to worry about tomorrow, and rest here. When that happens, it happens from sincerity. Faith is the only thing I know that defeats fear, and faith is found here in the breath. Beliefs are mind trappings, and faith is found outside the mind. Faith is not concerned with rationale, stories, or who did what; it is solely a place of devoting the heart to the gift of the present, then allowing the present to unwrap itself as it is, thus honoring unfolds. Faith knows nothing of proving (approval); it is simply is deep trust in the Divine now. This Divine is acknowledged in me honoring you, but I can't honor you fully unless I honor and accept my gift, which lies here. The gift of who I am is discovered moment-to-moment, breath-by-breath, and pose-by-pose.

We are not insignificant, lacking and limited, we are here, and that is enough. On my mat today I realized that I stand naked in my pose (not literally), using only what I have to give here. Each pose invites me to give more of myself, and it does not do it in a pushy, arrogant, holier than thou way, but it encourages me with grace, love, and gentleness. Today I fell and didn't care, and even laughed, because I can.

Andrew Harvey in his blog on *Walking the Christ Path through Life and Death Experience*, asks us to ponder these questions, and I leave you with them, "What did you do while the world was burning?" and "What did you love enough to really give your whole life for?"

Get your sweat on!

Day 7

"BEEP!"

Day seven of my 30 straight days of hot yoga at Moksha Los Angeles, and today before class I met the teacher Emily who suggested water; she handed me a bottle and talked to me about the importance of drinking water in the practice and the effects of dehydration. Thank goodness. Angels appear in all shapes and sizes and at the right times. What a blessing! I walked into class, lay down on my mat, and closed my eyes for about ten minutes. By the time class actually started I was a geyser of sweat; so thank goodness for the recommendation.

Today we focused on allowing the breath to fill the space in our bodies, directing the breath, and feeling it fill us up. I decided to add a challenge to my practice and really become a Jedi, yes a *Star Wars* reference. During some of the practice I closed my eyes, and found something very interesting: I seemed to trust my eyes, ears, and touch, more than my breath. Once I closed my eyes, I was wobbling, a little off, and had to sense alignment. Normally I can see it, or am guided to see it, go to it, but with my eyes closed, well everything changed. First, any story I was telling myself went out the window, because when you close your eyes you have no time to trust the mind; it is useless, and you realize how much of your mind relies on the senses for its information. So now my eyes were closed and it felt as if there was no body, with this vast undiscovered place, I felt like a tight ropewalker. I began to give way to the space Emily was talking about and sensed the greatness of the inner world. Wow! How much do I rely on my sight, sound, touch, taste, and smell to give me information that is only partially true.

So what is behind this mask I am wearing, behind my identities? Well like super heroes, or a Jedi master, I discovered that the inner world is vast and all my trust is there. But I have been conditioned to trust the senses (mind), and yet when I trust that it fails to hit the mark. An image came to me in my practice; many people suggest that "sin" is missing the mark. What is the mark we are missing? If the mark is happiness, love, bliss, or light, then our thoughts are the arrows. The invisible is the bow. So in the invisible I have a choice to let go of the thoughts (arrows), and when I let them go, they can be fearful thoughts, which I believe we all know, or as we dive into the inner world, we discover, can be love. Love always hits its mark. But love is an inner experience coming out; the mind is an outer experience coming in. Do you see? Once I left the mind, and began to dwell in the inner, then I could use my bow to shoot from the heart. Thus I could hit the mark correctly. How can I change my shot, if my shot is off, missing the mark? I go to the Divine with a sincere heart and I ask for help, forgiveness, or guidance. With sincerity comes the answer. Only in sincerity can we actually receive what we are asking.

My teacher Emily, today, seems to have a sincere way of teaching, and guiding us into our breath and inner world. I came up with the word "BEEP" or Be Energy Expressing Poses – I will work on it…onward to day eight…

Yoga and Yoda?

Later today I will be on day eight, but an idea occurred to me this morning as I watched the day begin. My day normally begins with my cat poking my face for food, so I don't need an alarm clock to wake up for my private time with God, which is meditation and listening. I took on this process of 30 days of straight yoga to offer myself a challenge; now at the time it was just that, to challenge me. But this morning I had the image of yoga being like Yoda from the *Star Wars* film series. Yoda was a character that Luke met, and who trained him. For when you are ready, the teacher will appear. Well that is what happened here, in my life.

When I first started taking yoga, I took it as a way of dealing with life and getting back in shape. As some of you have read in the early blogs, I came to it with a health challenge. Then as my practice grew stronger, I kept it up for physical reasons, which I felt was the natural flow or progression. Then that period wore off, and now I want to experience yoga from the mental, body, and spiritual place, which I am finding as I explore a deeper and richer inner life. The difference is that when I studied for over four years at Agape International Spiritual Center and became a practitioner, I was doing that at the time, to understand my own inner unhappiness. I was not happy inside. I was blessed to have teachers, ministers, and friends who to this day truly love me and care about me. I am truly honored by those relationships. And honored by my time here as well. A lot has shifted since my time in school.

But I recognize that the journey here is much different today. In school I was still coming from a conditional place of learning; meaning I read tons of books, did the work, was a good student, but it never reached my heart, though it hovered, and had its moments. The work came from being accepted, approved, and proving that I was good enough.

The difference today and going through this journey with you and opening up, is that I am ready to really learn. And yoga now is much different, fun, and filled with so much to learn. It isn't just some earthly practice without the spirit. I find that my practice now is listening: "The teacher has appeared and I am ready." My stubborn will doesn't work anymore, it used to work great as a way of motivating me in my craft as an actor, an "I'll show you, or you don't think I can do it," kind of language. But that motivation came from proving, and approval, which have nothing to do with love. Those are disguised resentments that I re-sent over and over to motivate me. Now my poses are teaching me and I am listening.

Day 8

"Yoga is Your Story"

It is day eight of 30 straight days of hot yoga at Moksha Yoga with teacher Joe. Years ago I dated a girl named Amanda who bought me a ticket to see Wayne Dyer speak. It would be the first time I would see him talk live in person. Upon entering the lobby, I noticed all the merchandise, books, etc…and after wandering around for a few moments, a lady announced, "Take your seats Dr. Dyer will be speaking soon."

At the box office some people were upset because the event was sold out. I stood and watched it all transpire, then I felt a wonderful energy stand right next me and speak to the group that was upset, it was Dr. Dyer and he said calmly, "Everyone will get in, we will make room for everyone." The chaos and drama all fell away, and that was that.

Tonight's practice was like that for me. I lay down on my mat, closed my eyes, and whispered a prayer: "Dear God, bless my practice, and whatever you reveal to me, let me accept it, be with it, and not judge it. Amen." And then the Wayne Dyer story flooded my heart: "Everyone will get in." Then like clockwork, teacher Joe explained to us before we started, "As a teacher or guide, yoga is up to you, it is about you, you breathing into those places, breathing into space, and finding strength and peace. Yes! Can you find the strength and peace in the pose?" Yoga welcomes everyone equally, just like the breath. The breath connects us all to each other. Judgment disconnects us from the breath. When I breathe without effort into the pose, it opens space and strength, and peace is natural, because there is no resistance to what is. The moment I begin to think, my breath stops and I fall. I am a not good thinker, because I am a breather who functions in being, and being is listening. Breathing and listening are active and engaging. So what I notice in my practice is, the more I allow the breath to take over my practice, the more I enter strength and peace in the heart, and can express myself physically. I find that if I begin to think, *this pose is difficult, or my God it's hot in here, or what are they doing?* I fall. Now there is nothing wrong with falling. When you are allowing the breath to guide you deeper, you go past what you know, and you fall. Then you get up and do it again.

A baby never just gets up when they are learning to walk, they find balance, fall over, and laugh at themselves. What I noticed with the practice tonight is what our teacher Joe suggested, "Yoga is your story revealing itself, and tonight is just a paragraph of it." I like that. It's gentle. Every day I show up on my mat, open my book and read the adventure of my heart, and discover a little bit more of myself in the pose. Sometimes it is wobbly, sometimes it is happy, and sometimes it is expressing itself with a big smile, but like life, the pose passes away, and the next one comes up. I find that in my practice when I allow, then "Everyone is welcome, and I make room." Who is everyone? They are the noise in my mind, the aches in the body, and the breath itself; it is all welcomed and then let go. Each breath welcomes the pose and lets it go. I will incorporate that in my life. The mat imitates life.

Day 9

"Yoga is Divine"

Well day nine of 30 straight days of hot yoga at Moksha Los Angeles found me with a more gentle approach. We flowed in the first half of the practice and then went in to restorative poses in the second half. Again, before practice, as I closed my eyes on my mat, I sat allowing the breath to flow uninhibited, meaning can I allow the breath to just flow easily through and out my body without resistance from the mind. This is what came forward, besides endless amounts of sweating. Yes, it is possible to allow the flow of breath and allow it to flow uninhibited by thoughts. It takes practice, and it is where I place my attention.

What I noticed was, when I place my focus on the mind, I push through aggressively and the pose becomes more like an animal and less like unity. But on the other hand, when I put my attention on the breath, I notice that the breath gracefully pushes me out, and the mind follows the breath. When the mind controls the practice the breath is very constrictive and tight; rather like when I got asthma as a kid. My chest tightens and I would gasp for air. The breath is life, and in some spiritual practices and religions it is acknowledged as the spirit. The bridge between heaven and earth is right here.

Yoga is divine. It is the connection between the earth and the heavens, which is what we need in our life: the balance of life. But as always it starts with our walk. We live in a society created by our unconscious agreements and conscious agreements, our stories bring us closer to each other, and rather than judge people, which is an easy way out of life, let us yearn to understand each other and by understanding we become closer to the Divine within and out. Just like Moksha Yoga is teaching me, it is my job when I practice to understand who I am in each pose.

Then by understanding myself, I can adjust accordingly. The same applies with people, if we can understand each other, then we can adjust accordingly.

Day 10

Blinded by the Light

Well folks as I move into day 10 of 30 straight days of hot yoga at Moksha Los Angeles, to say that today I gracefully entered my mat would be far from the truth. At home, I awaited my babysitter, then drove to yoga, rather than walk. Yes, as many of you know, I am a single dad, and there are many good dads out there and I hope you are recognized and celebrated; I know I am. Dads most times get a bum wrap, even when they are good. With that said, in yesterday's practice we went deep into our bodies, so my right hip was pretty much yelling at me today – and this was a wonderful opportunity to be with it. My practice today was a practice of being with it, and at one point the teacher acknowledged that we all have "sensations." I like that view. Once he said that I was able to be with the sensation in my hip, and be gentle with myself. As we moved along in the practice it started to lessen, and I could move through it. Once you observe something, it changes, so once I observed the sensations in my hip, it allowed me to move. I didn't deny it, or act like it wasn't happening. I just said YES to it!

As I move into the first third of 30 days completed, I find it has moved fast, and I have enjoyed the feedback from everyone. It seems to be helping people, which is wonderful. Moksha is wonderful community, of conscious men and women, and I am honored to be sharing my insights. If you get a chance and want to give hot yoga a try, I would recommend it. Move past the sweating part. Just because you sweat it doesn't mean you are working hard, the sweating is a great way to detox the body. One of the things I have learned from all the teachers in Los Angeles Moksha is the focus on the breath. Allowing the breath to guide the practice and giving your minds a break. Today we looked in the mirrors at our poses and I had my shirt off, talking about being blinded by the light, jeez.

I am going to take a warm shower now and go on to some play dates with my daughter.

Day 11

Yoga of Sincerity

It is day 11 of 30 straight days of hot yoga at Moksha Los Angeles. Today I entered practice, changing classes at the last minute, which worked out well. Something occurred in my practice that I would like to share. When I am truly present on my mat, then anticipation goes away, thinking slows down, and trust shows up. When we trust our teachers it comes from sincerity. We are sincere in learning, sincere in growing, and that sincerity brings about trust in the relationship. We then have openness to learning. If we lack trust, or have trust issues with others or ourselves, we don't listen fully, in fact we think about the next thing to say, or what we have to do, or we search for approval, or try to prove ourselves. So while on the yoga mat for 11 days I have noticed sincerity in my practice and in my life.

Once, when a friend of mine prayed, a transformation happened in his life. He had prayed for an answer and he received it quickly. We talked about how the transformation happened, when the other times he had prayed, he had received nothing, it seemed. We arrived at sincerity. His heart was sincere to receive and listen. It wasn't about knowing the answer, having more money, or attracting something. It was truly asking from a place of sincerity, because he had sincerely wanted to know. I have noticed people in my life that question not from a sincere place, but one of lack of trust of people and themselves. They want to build up more defenses towards being "special," and are looking to be right. I would much rather be happy than right as I get older.

Today with our teacher Kate guiding the practice, I asked a question about a pose I was in. She came down to meet me where I was and demonstrated with gentleness and care a new way to be with it. The adjustment helped me out tremendously and I was happy to receive the guidance. I thanked her at the end of class and she even explained that lots of people had been doing that and then shared with me some more on how it benefited my practice with the slight change. Trust is sincere. Being on my mat is about sincerity with each pose and being able to gently let them go, and being able to accept the next pose fully.

I have noticed in my life that I am developing more sincerity for life. I recognize that there are many people who are hurt, wounded, and in shame, so they may lash out, yell, or bully; but I am noticing that really they are calling out for love. Most people are calling out for love. On the mat we are calling in love and calling in our connection to the beloved within each of us. Every love story starts with sincerity and goes from there. Sincerely thank you for stopping by...on to day 12...

Day 12

"Tears in Heaven"

Day 12 of 30 straight days of hot yoga at Moksha Los Angeles, and after a couple of days of slowing down, today the theme song of Rocky could have been playing while I practiced, "Getting Strong Now." In all seriousness I felt very disciplined, alive, and strong on my mat. Our teacher Joe mentioned that the "breath moves through everything." I liked that. The breath is quite strong and does move through everything. The breath relaxes the body and the mind: pretty cool.

I did something today that I hadn't tried before, and there was a major part of my practice that was moving like a wild fire, fierce focus, fierce love, with my heart expressing outwards. What I tried was picturing my lungs as my nose; what I mean is, placing my attention on my lungs and breathing in through my lungs and out through them. It felt great, and deep and profound. I could feel my ribs really expand as though they were catching the full breath and then letting it go. The breath drove my practice. I really just let it rip today. No holding back. At the tail end of my practice I really dove into my hips, and felt how expansive I felt in them. A couple of days ago, they were tight and now they were alive and willing.

Today I was alive and willing. Three years spent holding back, not being heard, not being seen, was no fault of anyone but me. So for that I forgive. I never really saw myself, heard myself, embraced myself, congratulated myself, I was too busy helping others live, and some people take advantage of that. Today that aspect of me – the side not heard, seen, embraced – burned up under this full moon. Enough is enough. Have you ever felt that way? Have you ever just said "screw it," dropped everything and went for it?

Today was that day. I love being a dad, and my next-door neighbor said to me, as her grandson and my daughter played, "David, you are a really loving dad, you are great with Harper, she is going to really fly because of you."

I smiled and said, "Thank you I appreciate that."

Then there was a beat in the conversation, the type of beat that lets you know something from the heart is coming, and out of the pause came this: "David, you'll find the right woman, she will see you, she will, you're a catch." I took it in, and said, "Thank you."

On my mat today, I really caught who I am. Joe our teacher mentioned, "Freedom is in choice." I chose freedom tonight. After class, I walked home, and felt strong, and tall, alive, and open. The sky was blue, with clouds, and sunlight finding its way through. I cried. I just cried. No reason, just healing, just loving myself again. Nothing to fix, nothing to change, just tears, letting go. Feeling. Feeling the power of my heart. Feeling the beloved. On to day 13... Sweat on!

Day 13

"Respect Your Temple"

Day 13 of 30 straight days of hot yoga at Moksha Los Angeles, and as I entered the yoga studio I was informed that Lululemon Athletic Yoga gear has invited me to share my blog on their social media sites. So thank you for that!

Today our teacher Joe reminded us of our body temples and respecting them. Two things popped in my mind, the first was traveling around Montreal years ago and walking into an old 1800s cathedral and looking up at the vastness of it. I have no words now and had no words then, just "AWE." The second was my own temple. On either side of our forehead we our have left and right temples. As we close our eyes we enter our temple. By placing our attention in the center of the head, we rest in the one eye, the one heart, and the one breath. Now keeping your attention in the center of your head will drop your eyelids half way, and you may look like a Buddhist master but this is being in the center of your temple. In the center of your head, look out through your own eyes, you will notice the mind has stopped, and you are in your temple.

So I began practice today respecting my temple, being gentle, resting in its vastness and AWE and sitting in the center of it. Since I started the 30 days, some subtle things have shifted – eating watermelon, apples, grapes, mango, and fruits, and savoring the taste, and drinking just one cup of coffee in the morning, the rest of the time water. And there are other changes in my mental and emotional life as well. I am experiencing kindness with myself, watching my language, respecting people even when they seem different, wanting to understand more, and forgiving a lot more.

I went through a tough three years with some people who

were very cruel and unkind. I had a lot of resentment, anger, and unkindness in my temple that I carried around like a cross. Then I realized that resentment wants my way to be right and their way to be wrong, and they probably thought they were right and I was wrong. Silly I know, but that is where I was, until one day, after being in my temple in silence, a question came to me: "David, do you want to happy or right?" I thought, "Happy." So I had to let go of all the places where I wanted to be right, and replace them with happy. There is a wonderful saying, "Just because you're right doesn't mean I am wrong." I like that, wonderful reminder.

So the final thing that came up on my mat today was what are the rules of my temple? Well the same rules that are brought up in my practice. Here are the rules, breathe. Just let the breath guide the temple. The heart is the altar, and as we sit at the altar, to alter our perspective, we allow the breath to be the guide as we inquire within, "How do I treat others?" Well we breathe the same air, and since I honor my breath, I honor your breath and you. Simple.

Day 14

"Are You Disturbed?"

So I came into day 14 of 30 straight days of hot yoga at Moksha Yoga, and before practice I lay on my mat and closed my eyes; and as I lay there I noticed something. Here I am lying down and breathing, simple, right? Yet what changes when I get on my feet in a pose and start moving? Yes, the room is hot; yes, there are people everywhere; yes, the poses flow. But what is changing this peace of mind that I am experiencing on my mat as I lay here now? So I wondered if I could find out. Well if you look, you will find. If you ask, it is given. In all religions, and spiritual practices when you look at the core teachings, they all have some common ground; like all yoga practices the breath is common, and in all customs, religions, and spiritual practices, "Be still." So what disturbs your peace of mind? Piece of our mind tries to disturb our peace of mind.

As I moved into the pose and was breathing and allowing the breath in, I noticed that the mind would react to it (The Physical), and the reactive mind would disturb my peace of mind. So I began to witness with the breath breathing the pose, and I watched the mind create an interpretation of what may be going on. But as I listened to the mind interpret the pose, its logic was so far from the truth. I began to see the irrational mind at work. As I witnessed the pose, and would just breathe with it, the mind would dive in loudly, like a scared child, and panic: "This is impossible, you can't do this, you will fall, look bad, oh my goodness, nooooo!" I listened with the breath and saw that the mind was seeing the pose, and by seeing it, was outside of it. But when I was breathing into the pose I would pass the mind-programmed drama, which put me into the pose, inside myself, and from there falling down became playful, fun, and childlike, not childish. This is a big breakthrough for myself and I hope I am explaining this correctly for you.

The mind is attached to the body sensations and from there creates an identity of drama, chaos, joy, etc...depending on thoughts; but the breath when I am fully engaged in it, creates peace, strength, and allows for a deeper practice. From the vantage point of the breath I am the witness, and from this place, I am allowed to be childlike, in wonder, and laugh more, and be playful; but when I choose to engage the mind I notice I become strict, judgmental, suffocated, and falling down is a shot to approval.

I learn more when I am relaxed, loose, playful, and having fun. When the intellect gets too involved, I become like a serious robot and want to show off in my pose. But yoga isn't about how flexible you are, it is about many other things, but for me it shows you what disturbs your peace of mind in every pose. So what disturbs your peace of mind?

Midpoint

"Where is the switch?"

Later today I will be entering my 15th day of 30 straight days of hot yoga at a wonderful studio and community in Los Angeles called Moksha Yoga.

I was talking to my daughter's teacher about this challenge of 30 straight days and some of my insights, and she was very encouraging. She said, "Good for you!"

I was listening to a teacher the other day giving a talk on relationships, and the importance of positive encouragement. For example, men love to hear from their partners, "I am proud of you, I know how hard you are working, or I know you didn't get so and so, but I am so proud of you, and what you bring to this world every day." And on the other hand, men need to encourage their wives, or partners, with the same positive reinforcement, such as, "You are so beautiful today, or thank you for all you do for our family, or you look great, or I love your laugh, I am so blessed by you," etc... I was reminded of this when I heard my daughter's teacher compliment me. There is a lot of telling, fixing, changing, and not a lot of meeting people where they are, and respecting them, cheering them on, not wanting anything in return, just because love gives love. And because when we meet people, we see their divinity and honor them. You may judge me for example, but if I know who I am, then I still see you as love, and know you are caught in your mind. Why? – because I have been there too, and I realize that it is painful place to be. And I listen and bless you inwardly. This is the practice, everyone is our teacher, and we are learning to be the fullest expression of who we are.

As I enter my midpoint on this 30-day challenge, I realized that I had spent most of my life looking for the switch in the dark.

Whether that was called enlightenment, awakening, love, or even light. Having this big moment when I get "it." So I took many classes, studied with some of the best teachers, did workshops, read tons of books, counseled, spoke, wrote, meditated, prayed, all with the sense of getting something, some moment, that was already here. Yes I have grown, yes it has been a wonderful ride, and continues to be, yet now, I find doing these 30 days of hot yoga to be a practice of being with it, whatever comes up.

Be with the breath, with the pose, with life, and allow the rational mind to surrender itself. Yoga is a practice. A practice of arriving here, dancing with the nature of life, and yes life offers you strength like mountain pose, twists in the spine like the struggles of relationships or jobs, flipping life over and seeing it differently like in back bends, seeing things differently by standing on your head, and of course in the Corpse pose. Yoga has taught me and continues to teach me that the mat is life. We start in Child pose and we go through 40 postures to end on our mat in Shavasana. Like life, yoga offers us, the benefit of being with our growth, our learning, and our presence. Our life is experienced in 60, 75, or 90 minutes on the mat. Then, like life, the thrill, excitement, drama, or whatever you choose to experience in each pose, is gone in a flash. But in the moment of it, it can feel like a long minute – a really long minute of breathing into it – and I am honored by this journey, and hope this journey is honoring you as well. So I ask, "Where is the switch?" I sense the switch is when you can see clearly in the dark. Reminder, all things end, all things have cycles, like your breath. This too shall pass! Love you.

On to day 15 today SWEAT ON!

Day 15

Halfway Home

Wait for it! Day 15 of 30 straight days of hot yoga at Moksha LA, and wow, it went very fast indeed. Halfway home. Today I lay on my mat and had a tough time concentrating; so I figured the rest of my practice would be that way. So I lay there with my eyes closed and watched the mind wanting to pull my focus away from where I was, and frankly it was winning. The mind talked and I began to follow what I have been writing here on just following the breath, and as I did that, somewhere along the line, the mind was gone and I was firmly on my mat and in my practice.

When we began, a strange image passed by – the image of the turtle and the rabbit. In the moral tale, the rabbit sprints out, but at the end of the race, the turtle beats the rabbit. That is what I feel this journey has taught me: to be patient, breathe with it, and enjoy the poses or don't enjoy them. Either way you have to be with them as they are, and finally give yourself a break if you need it. I heard recently of some 40-year-old men dying of heart attacks. I bring this up not to be morbid, but sometimes, in my poses, my face is so serious as if the pose is life and death, and today I had that moment where I caught myself and smiled. Sometimes life is short and sometimes it's not, but however long it is for me, I would like to enjoy where I am, whether working, writing, school, life, or just being with where I am, and enjoying it.

This week I have felt very strong in my practice and the breath has really helped me dive deeper into the body and release the mind chatter. My goal was 30 days of hot yoga, and wow, as I said before, 15 days moves quickly. Well here is to the next 15 days, and I really appreciate all the support and feedback. I hope this is helping you too. Today a woman next to me was fanning herself because she was hot and I asked if she wanted my water, and she smiled and said, "I have some, thank you. Thank you for being so kind." We are a community of seven billion people, and it is time we came together for the planet, for life, and to help each other. Love is a giving energy and yoga gives us the opportunity to show up, be present, and expand to a bigger place; and it does it, like all things in nature, in its own time.

God bless you.

Day 16

"I Can"

I walked to Moksha studio this morning, ready and willing, as I approached day 16 of 30 straight days of hot yoga. As I lay on my mat, I connected to the breath, my body on the mat, and the space inside me. For the first time I moved from the back of the room to the front, resting there, feeling the breath move through the body.

In the silence of the room, our teacher entered. "Let's look at our practice as 'I can,'" she said. "You have a choice on how you experience this practice." So my intention was set, "I can." So many days of my life were wasted in "I can't"; well at least three years ago they were. Now I find myself in a process of change, it seems to happen every time I am on my mat, feeling my way through. Today was no different, living in each pose, relishing the breath, the pose, and expressing "I can." Feeling stronger now in my practice, I stood in the front row, and the mirror was right in front of me. I saw myself strong in the pose. It surprised me. Do you ever have moments in your life where someone sees you, and you think, "Well that can't be right"? Well seeing myself in the mirror, I saw my strength, I saw my eyes, I saw my life, and for the very first time. What surprised me was the way I had been thinking about self and now seeing myself was like seeing two different people.

Here, before me, was this strong, energized, capable, and incredible being; yet for so many years the whispers in my mind had been suggesting otherwise. I remember when I was married, and sitting at the restaurant and two family members gave my daughter a pink cheerleading dress, and suggested that I could wear it too. At the time I was a stay at home dad, busting my hump, working my tail off to take care of our daughter. Now I ask myself, what in the world were they looking at? Were they looking at their own reflections, the parts they were afraid to see, that were evident when we sat together? Who knows? But I saw a glimpse today of what others see when they see me. It made me smile. Have I made mistakes? Oh yes, we all have, it is part of growth, part of learning, but today I say, "I could, I can, I surrender to my bigger self, I trust the breath breathing me." Does this make sense? To see who you actually are? To really see yourself? Embrace it.

Maybe this is what love is, beloved looking back at itself. I like that. On to day 17... Love you.

Day 17

It's happening?

I am on day 17th of 30 straight days of hot yoga at Moksha Yoga Los Angeles. Today, when I lay down on the mat, I contemplated the intention for today, but all that came up, was "now." So rather than fight or figure out the meaning of this, a question followed: "It's happening?" – wait for it – "Now." Everything was happening now, and so I chose to embrace "now" as the poses came up. This may seem like a big "Duh!" for those practicing for many years, or maybe even some starting; but I feel in my practice that every day is meeting "now" as it is. Every day practicing yoga is a beginner day. Because I find that if it isn't then I would have closed off to the opportunity to grow and learn, and that would stink, because it would mean I am closed off to the opportunities of the mat.

Today our teacher Carolina set an intention for the class with releasing control, and it is funny in each pose how I try to control it: squeezing the toes, holding the jaw. In fact I have found in my life generally, that when I am holding on to something, I squeeze my toes and crunch them up. So today was a wonderful opportunity to embrace the ways in which I control a pose. As we explored the poses today, I found places where my body wanted to express in the upper back, and my mind was saying, "Um no you can't." So I would breathe, and let the breath expand me up through it. And you know what? I did it. I recognized that on a deeper level, everything is happening now and the mind is either rushing backwards or forward, to play ignorant to what is happening now. But if I can allow everything to rest here, the gains are incredible, the pose becomes its own expression, and I can feel freedom from the past and future, and the consistent negating of who I am or looking out and comparing outside to me.

As I have been practicing Moksha Yoga I have noticed the freedom in the breath, and the importance of embracing the pose as it is. It sounds simple and every teaching sounds simple in the intellect, until you walk it, breathe it, and live it. It is easy to be right, who cares; we are here to discover happiness within and without.

Day 18

"Where Did That Go?"

Well finishing off day 18 of 30 straight days of hot yoga at Moksha Yoga Los Angeles, and lying on my mat with my eyes closed, I was reminded of the day I went skydiving. As the plane climbed higher and higher in the air, my fear did too. I was strapped to the instructor and so I was going to jump. Fearful thoughts raced through my head as I sat at the edge of the plane looking out, two miles up in the air, feet dangling. The instructor said, "Okay, David, we have to jump now. Let's do it." I went, into the abyss, facing the fear head on, and the mind stopped, and we glided across the sky. It was awe-inspiring. No words can describe the feeling of jumping. The same holds true for yoga. Yes, the mind may be racing in a pose, yes, the mind may be trying to get your attention, but all you can do is breath into it, be with it, and allow the fearful thoughts to go. I learned and I am still learning that these thoughts are just defending us, and protecting us, from what? Who cares? It just becomes endless stories on stories.

Today my practice felt like jumping out of the plane. Was my mind racing? Not too much, but my breath and heart wanted to move past what they knew, they wanted to go deeper and express. The heart was ready to be the leader and the breath was ready to use her grace. Karma means, "come back." So how we treat others and ourselves comes back to us. Everything on the mat comes back to you; and yet in stillness and quiet within, there is no karma. Crazy but true. Yoga is an invitation to meet your life on your mat, and no one can push you, or tell you where you should be. It is entirely up to you, to make the commitment to follow the breath, the heart, and jump.

I have learned many valuable lessons in practicing Moksha.

One is the breath is so important; two, that falling is okay, and when I say fall, just fall over; and three, the breath will help you find alignment and alignment is very important. Take time. Enjoy the class. Enjoy the poses. Meet the pose right where I am today. Be willing to be willing. Listen. The breath is your friend. Yoga is your friend. The pose is your friend. The mat is the space of safety, security, and comfort, and you will not be harmed, or hurt. So in the safety of your mat, relax onto it and experience you fully. Your body is your temple, so respect it. Life is happening now. When I truly honor myself on the mat, then I can fully honor you.

Day 19

Yoga is Rebellious

So I came into day 19 of 30 straight days of hot yoga at Moksha. Walking in I felt exhausted, tired, and lay down on my mat. Each day that I lay on my mat, it feels a womb, safe, secure, and a place to be who I am. It is a place to embrace every aspect of who I am. Frankly I can let it be. Teacher Joe is a wonderful guide back inside for many, including myself. I appreciate his guidance, his words, and his music selection.

Off my mat, I realize so many people have expectations they put on you, and in fact I had met a friend earlier in the day, and as I walked into the cafe, one of the employee's saw me come in and commented, "Man, you look great, what are you doing?"

I said, "30 straight days of hot yoga, I am on day 19 today."

He replied with a smile, "Cool, keep it up."

As I turned to walk away, another woman asked the gentlemen in a whisper, "What is he doing? Oh that sounds horrible." I wanted to turn back and reply, "Your inner voice is speaking out." But I listened and felt in my body the sensations one feels as a kid, when some other kid announces to the others, "Where did he come from?"

I find that my practice on my mat is life – my life – and that there is no difference, as it keeps pointing me inward. As Joe said in class, "The breath can be used in your life when you want to relax, breathe deep a couple times, and let it relax you." Today I had moments of wobbling, and strength, and grace, and sweat, and in one funny moment I caught myself in the mirror and said, "Wow I really do think I look like Casper the Friendly Ghost with my shirt off." This practice every day has become a Godsend, a gift, because it gives me some sanity in a world pushing me to be like everyone else. I feel as if when someone finds the mat, they are ready to experience who they really are, with no BS, and no excuses. And in my life, I was tired of running like Forrest Gump. Tired of taking things so seriously, exhausted with approval, proving, and trying to be something. What I have always craved for is knowing who I am – really am. Not the intellectual. Not the label. Not the box people seem to put you in such as, "Oh David is divorced." Or the box I agree to put myself into, to fit in. But to know my BIG SELF.

Today, after 19 days of straight yoga, I began to find my strength and I stood on my hands from Tree pose on both sides. A little victory, to say, "Yes, world, I matter. I can. I am. I will." Of course ten minutes later in Shavasana I wept, let it all go, surrendered, stopped resisting, and lay there in my sweat, my tears on my mat – laying myself open. It was then I wished that I had someone to hold me, so I could be heavy in her arms. I used to see tears as weakness, but now I see tears as great strength, just like forgiveness. Only the strong can forgive. Only the strong can love without fear.

Yoga is rebellious because the world is attached to the body, and the mind as identifiers, and yoga says, "This is not who you are, you are not worry, you are more, or rather 'amore' love." It takes a real rebel to turn from the mind and body and stand in the breath, like a rock, in stillness, when the world inside you is telling you otherwise – that is real rebellion. And as you stand in your breath, on your mat, with sweat, sensations, mind chatter, and body positions, and say I accept this as it is, then that is rebellious. You can't hide on your mat and you can't hide in life. Yoga is rebellious!

Day 20

Yoga is Unity

Well here I am, day 20 of 30 straight days of hot yoga at Moksha Yoga Los Angeles, and as I lay on my mat before class, I brought my attention to different parts of my body. To my feet, my legs, my abs, my shoulders, my head, and I noticed by simply bringing awareness to my feet for example, without changing them, they relaxed. Suddenly my body temple was grounded on the mat, eyes closed, and everything was relaxed. It felt lovely to lay there; my throat felt sore, but that was okay. But I noticed a presence that was alert, calm, and ready. So I decided what would be in my practice today would be that alert presence.

Joe our teacher entered the room and discussed with us many reminders, but one in particular was that the breath is powerful, and that yoga is sustained through the breath, through the inside out. The practice is within – out. The expression is from within, and then comes the physical. As we moved through our practice today I noticed this alertness, awareness in each pose, and it seems to notice and adjust in the presence without effort; but when my mind is engaged in the pose, I become willful and push it. I then became aware of two movements within my practice, one subtle and quiet, and the other loud and pushy. Now the thing that helped me when I recognized the pushy part was first becoming aware of it, and then breathing with it, and then alignment comes. I was in the Down Dog pose and my shoulders intuitively went back and in, I was aligned. It felt great. The discovery today of this alert presence led to something quite wonderful towards the end of practice. We had closed our eyes and Joe our teacher wanted us to feel the breath in the body, and suddenly I became aware of the power of the breath and the fragility of the body.

The breath moving down to the hips and the stomach expands like elastic; the ribs expand, and out through the nose. It really is quite extraordinary and this powerful process goes on unconsciously for most people; but to feel it and recognize the fragility and the strength of the body temple was amazing. Someday my body will feed the earth, the spirit will add itself back in to the air, and my mind will go with the body. Yet I have the opportunity everyday on my mat and off my mat to unify the body, mind, and spirit as one. That is wonderful news. I have that opportunity in my practice to unify the mind, the body, and spirit – awesome! And the foundation, the practice is allowing the powerful breath to move through and do its work. That is faith to be still, when all around you is in chaos, and to listen, just listen.

Day 21

Rise and Shine

Well here I am at 4:30 am, warm in my bed, and my alarm clock is going off. Day 21 of 30 straight days of hot yoga finds me going to the 6 am class. Today is busy and to keep up with the 30 straight days of hot yoga, 6 am was the only time I could fit in. After getting up, I walked down to the studio, entered, lay my mat down, and closed my eyes. I probably could have slept but felt really good that my discipline, focus, and passion are back in my life. Yoga has given me purpose. My intention for my blog when I started was to show that each of us can make a difference by changing ourselves, and that change can be difficult. Now I will admit, the world can be a little crazy with wars, news, abuse against women and children, greed, etc...but it starts with us. So what can I do? I can get on my mat and deal with things with an open mind. I used to think that if you worried, you cared about people, but now I understand that worry is a curse on people, and it gets no one anywhere and makes things worse. It is bad karma. To arrive at that understanding I had to discover it within myself.

Yoga allows me the opportunity to discover who I am? What I am? And that is powerful, challenging, and also can be lots of fun. Today our teacher Joe explained that as you trust more, you flow more. I am finding that within my practice I trust the breath, and the feeling with it. Listening to the body, and allowing the breath to flow into the space of the aches, pains, sorrows, disappointments, failures, success, abundance, etc...I am aware this life on the mat is a wonderful as it teaches us about walking the walk. For as I learn on my mat, I take it into life and apply it.

What does walking the walk mean? Simply showing up and speaking from your heart, being open, honest, and knowing that your word means something, honoring yourself and others, and seeing their divinity and yours. See? Not easy. Now we know why it is the road less traveled. Who wants to be in pain, hurt, and yet that is the invitation. To keep opening up and trusting the flow of life, even as things are ending.

After my divorce, I closed down my heart, closed down the flow, and treated myself unkindly inwardly with words, and so when others started treating unkindly I took it. I was so use to the inward punishment, I felt I deserved it. I felt like a failure, I felt lots of stuff that I didn't feel safe expressing. I wanted to be strong for my daughter, be strong for my audience, put on a good show, a good face, and act as though I could handle it. I did sometimes, but most days I was not good. Now I am coming up and rising. Thank goodness. There is something bigger.

I had to go through that time in my life to teach me, to help me see who I am today, to bless those in my life, to forgive, to learn to really love, and to let go of the conditional and open up. To me, that is real strength, not putting people down, or having power over people, or control, or judgment; those are tools to keep us closed off. So yes today I rise and shine. Opportunities abound. A new life is here and I am honored by the love of my family for their support, to my friends for their support, and to the biggest inspiration on the planet and my teacher my daughter Harper. Remember you can always hit restart, wherever you are.

Two Classes in One Day, "YIN"

Yes, you read it right, day 21 of 30 straight days of Moksha Yoga, found me ending my night with Yin. It is a slow, mindful practice that works into your deep tissue. Waking up at 4:30 am today for the 6 am class, I was inspired to end my night in the Moksha practice of Yin. I am glad I did. My day was swamped with lots of activities, which is good, but sometimes when I am swamped with activities I forget to take care of myself and honor myself at the end of the night. I am learning how to be gentle with myself, honor my life now, and rest with things, not in a passive way, just in a place of mindfulness. Many people on this planet are striving for a goal, pushing things, controlling things, and the Yin practice is complete surrender to now. The poses are designed so that you rest in them, and breathe deeply. There were a couple of them we held and I was surprised by the acceptance I had. As the sensations in certain parts of my body were screaming for attention, I brought my breath into them and felt the quiet, surrender of each one. Following my breath, as it sensually dove into the sensations of the body, it felt like grace diving deep into the ocean.

Emily our teacher was a wonderful guide, reminded us of now, with affirmations, "I breathe in the breath, I breathe out the breath." I have had moments lately in my life, where it feels as if angels are speaking through people, and there is a wonderful knowing that shines from Emily. I really felt like in the Yin practice of yoga that it was time to rest, honor, and feel me from the inside out – very soothing. I met some people before class, who were very inspiring to be around – a wonderful community of heart-centered beings at Moksha. It feels wonderful to be around uplifting people, who are discovering who they are, and I am excited by the possibilities of this new beginning.

Yin practice allowed my walk home to be one of blessings and thanksgiving. I thought of my parents, and what an honor to move on this path of bigger love and teach each other about love, and their support is much appreciated. To my sister for showing me fierce love, fierce compassion, and to speak up. To Christine for all the support, friendship, energy, and prayers. To Rose for always shining her light on the planet and on me. To Candy for her willingness and grace and her walking it. To John for his support no matter what happens and his new life. To Liz, a constant source of power, big love, and clarity on situations and life. To Eric and Rose for being a vessel of learning, and growing as a couple and individuals. To Kristi who works so hard, and shines her light by allowing us on Patheos to shine, by the way we are seen. To Korena, for her healing energy and soon to be released book. To Renee my ex, may the blessings of life and the good of God light your way. To my daughter Harper, you are my light, my love, and my teacher; I am blessed you decided to come into my life and open me up to my worth, when for so long I felt unworthy. To Theresa, Matt and Lily may the new baby be blessed and loved. To Joe at Moksha, thank you for supporting my blog and passing it on, and teaching me in my practice that life is connecting to the breath. To Melanie, sometimes we come into situations that seem to want us to run back to our comfort, but you are a light and may you keep going forward. Steve Allen, thank you for seeing me as a speaker, writer, and friend: blessings on your family.

May you remember that you make a difference in someone's life, we all do, and when you give freely without wanting anything, it comes back to you in ways you can hardly ever imagine. God bless you and your families, partners, friends, and children. We are one. On to day 22…

Day 22

Petty Mind, Graceful Breath

How wonderful is this life? Really good. Those of you just joining me for the first time, I am approaching day 22 of 30 straight days of hot yoga at Moksha Yoga Los Angeles. I wrote my blog with the intention of diving deeply into my heart and discovering the strength in vulnerability. Throughout the last 22 days, I have been sharing my insights, struggles, and inspirations, and how yoga on and off my mat is the same.

In the process, I have surrendered the old life, and discovered the experience of her, the divine breath-heart, which I call Grace. She is the leader and power of my practice. When I started, I have to admit I was a little reluctant to trust her as I had trusted the pettiness of the mind for so long. But I have discovered her, the breath, sensual, alive, and strong, and her wisdom is amazing. She understands me, and quiets my pettiness, the parts that are scared, running, or escaping from the mat, she simple says, "Shhhh" as she quiets the child. Grace sounds like the tide in Santa Monica. She has taught me, to surrender to her, to stay grounded in her, and to respect her. She teaches me inside with intuition and guides me with ease into the next pose, not wanting me to look back, but fully trust her, trusting that I have fully honored "now" in the pose, that I have given my best, and now move forward.

Today our teacher Joe brought forth many instructions on trusting the breath, living in the breath, and going to the breath. It seems simple, but until you are on the mat practicing, you might not see how quickly the "pettiness comes in." The pettiness is concerned with everything that is not actually happening now. The pettiness on the mat is saying, "Hey, after class, I have to go to...or last night I can't believe...or look at their pose how amazing, or oh crap I can't do this." Then I remember her, Grace comes in. "Shhh listen, child, just listen to the breath." And you know what? The pettiness goes away. The attention goes back inside and all is well. She is good.

Now off my mat I am connecting with the breath more, listening to her, and trusting her.

Day 23

Giving Birth on the Mat

It is seven days away from my intention of 30 straight days of hot yoga at Moksha Yoga LA. I walked into day 23 with a newfound sense of trust. As I lay on my mat before practice I rested in the breath, knowing that the practice would be vigorous with Yang and would slow down in the Yin part. So I set the intention to go with the flow. As Robi entered the class he reminded us of the practice today, it would be strong, and then would end in the last half with holding poses longer.

As we started the practice I felt very strong in the poses, alive, and expressive. As we continued I noticed the mind wanting to get involved, but the breath would come in and relax me back into the pose. I noticed that the mind wanted to creep in when my body felt lots of sensations, or was tired, or while holding the pose for long periods of time. Recognizing those places in my practice, I can adjust by allowing the breath to flood those areas. I have been drinking water a couple of hours before each practice and that is making a huge difference both in my strength, my recovery, and peace of mind. Our teacher Rob really focused early on with the flow, and posture – moving with the breath and letting the breath guide us deeper on the mat.

As we entered the Yin practice of class, we held some poses in the hamstrings for long periods of time. I am noticing now how much better I am in holding the poses for longer, and my growing edge is actually in flowing in flow with the breath that seems to be a growing opportunity for my practice. Thank goodness it is just that, a practice, no need to worry about mastership, just show up on the mat, give your best, and breathe; oh yes, and sweat lots.

I recognize that on my mat, as I practice and blossom, that

each pose is a like a mini birth, and as I feel with it and with the sensations of the body, I begin to birth a new "me" – a "me" that can handle things, breathe with them, and relish peace of mind, rather than allowing the pettiness of the mind, or others, to disturb this inner peace.

Day 24

Transitions

I arrived at the studio and slipped into an earlier class. Trusting everything happens on time and in time. This is day 24 of 30 straight days of hot yoga at Moksha. I lay down on my mat and closed my eyes, relaxing my mind, and settling on my intention. I ended up sticking with my intention of going with the flow.

Emily, our teacher, entered the class wanting us to practice moving through transitions. So most of our transitions were slow and focused, and on moving from one pose to another, feeling the breath in the body, feeling the movement in them as we made our transitions. I have had the opportunity to deal with many different transitions, but as I rested in the movement of the transition of the pose, I recognized how sometimes I want to move through it and not want to be with it. But moving with it and allowing it to be as it is, was quite powerful. It allowed my breath to experience fullness, aliveness, and fluidity. When I pushed through the transitions I felt the breath speeding up or stopping, as if the breath was trying to put on the brakes, and say, "David we need to move with this."

Emily led us through the flow with the same intention, feeling the transitions, slowing it down, feeling the muscles work in each pose, and feeling how strong we are in the slowness. It was enjoyable to experience a new way of flowing in the practice, not pushing. Day 24 of 30 was wonderful to collect myself, slow it down, refine, redefine, and engage fully and slowly.

It is always a pleasure to be in a big class with people; it feels good to go through things with others, knowing we are going through the poses together, and yet we are supporting each other. How wonderful.

Day 25

Yoga is Divine

Well my day started in the valley giving a talk on faith, seeing fear as inverted faith, and then going to stand in it. Day 25 of 30 straight days of hot yoga at Moksha Los Angeles continued with another Yin practice. Yin practice is a practice designed for longer, deeper holds, and it helps you get into the tissue. When I arrived at the studio I placed my mat on the floor and lay down. I must have fallen asleep, because I awoke to my teacher's voice. Todays practice really focused on slowing it down, resting deeply in the breath, and taking our time. I noticed my jaw a lot – the tension there. So I was gentle in the class today with myself.

A lot of my gentleness was because of my growth in the practice and I had just talked at Unity Burbank. What is different is that normally I continue to give and give and give after a talk and by the end of the day I am exhausted. Today I gave and then lay back on my mat and received. It felt good to feel the giving and receiving. Sophie our teacher was wonderful and playful as she experienced the practice with us. We held some poses for up to five minutes and you could feel the stretching and breathing working together. I love discovering the community inside me.

I love the fact that in the morning I was called to be extraordinary and talk, then this afternoon in my practice I was called to be ordinary. The balance of the day has been wonderful and refreshing. The message in my talk and in this practice is the same, when fear comes it is a reminder to breathe with it, and as you breathe, and as you relax into the fear, you develop a new muscle – faith.

Faith for me is standing in peace of mind, undisturbed by the mind, body sensations. Peace of mind is my recognition of my connection to the Divine. The moment I leave peace of mind, I am separate, lost, confused, because I left my connection. I become a scared child, like any child would if they lost their parents. So yoga offers me a new way to connect to the Divine. By practicing being here now.

Day 26

"Oh Well"

I walked into day 26 of 30 straight days of hot yoga at Moksha, feeling a little off center. I entered the classroom and put my mat down, closed my eyes, and set the intention to just breathe consciously in each pose. Simple? Well maybe not so much tonight. Actually my intention would have been well served by smiling, and laughing more, because that is what happened. Our teacher Sophie offered us a Moksha practice that allowed us freedom to fall, be gentle, but not a practice to get angry with ourselves. Sophie explained anger tenses the body and we are here to let that go. My daughter is five and half now, when she was three, she used to drop lots of drinks and food on the floor. This happened quite a bit.

My daughter is my teacher and teaches me quite a bit about the presence of love as father. So one day she dropped some juice, and I said, "Oh well." It just came out. Then my daughter said, "Oh well, Dad." And then I said, "Every time we spill, we will say 'Oh well,' then clean it up, sound good?" She agreed.

I bring this lesson I learned from my daughter up, because tonight's practice was wobbly, and as I was in it, I heard, "Oh well." I smiled. What can you do but do your best now, right? The rest takes care of itself.

Yoga practice has taught me to smile more, breathe, and if you fall, get right up and do it again. Life is a practice. So we practice every day. We have moments where we judge, gossip, criticize, condemn, or get into someone's business, when we shouldn't be there. We recognize it, forgive it, and move on. Simple. Life is happening. Sometimes things work, sometimes they don't. Or we say, "Oh well I goofed up, it happens." Life is a practice of loving ourselves, and loving and honoring ourselves in the other as well.

Day 27

The Diamond Discovery

So I am inching closer, one breath at a time, as I approach day 27 of 30 straight days of hot yoga at Moksha. Today as I lay on my mat, with my eyes closed, and I had an image of a diamond. It was shiny, strong and beautiful. In the diamond was me, and as I looked at it closer, I saw all of us shining. In yoga practice we are offered the opportunity to connect to our inner diamond. Some of us have been away from it for so long that we feel time has passed. It has not. The beauty of the inner diamond is that it is always awaiting us to acknowledge it, trust it, and then shine it out.

Today's practice guided by Melanie was a chance to shine and acknowledge our inner diamond, and marvel at the magnificent life we are. She reminded us how one bead of sweat forms on our body and of all the millions of cells working for that to happen. Our bodies are green sustainable energy. How wonderful to come inside and acknowledge our beauty inward. I love gratitude and the real feeling of it. Not gratitude to get more stuff, but gratitude for all that is here now. It makes my heart smile.

Each of us has gone through crap. Unhealthy people, unhealthy relationships, jobs, criticism, money – we have been on both ends of the spectrum. But sooner or later, we must acknowledge that none of it is who we are. Did it happen? Yes, but through it all the diamond was shining. Everything, everybody, and every situation was and is working for us, getting us close to the diamonds we are inside. Inviting us in gently. So let's celebrate us, be kind to us, and "us" means you and I connected to one another.

Forgiveness takes great strength sometimes, because the hurts pile up, and some people seem to love sending hurts to others.

Here is the kicker, when you don't forgive and let go, both of you play tug of war with each other. Proving, being right, and making the other wrong, but there is no winner, sometimes jobs, relationships, run their course, and we are called to move upward and let go. So when we forgive, we let go of our end of the rope, and walk away. We can create a new story, a new path, and get closer to the diamond. I open to receive new possibilities in work, travel, speaking jobs, relationship and so forth, that is for the good of all and doesn't hurt anyone.

On to day 28...

Day 28

Wrestling with Yourself

I approached day 28 of 30 straight days of hot yoga at Moksha, and as I walked to the 6 am class, I found I was arguing with myself, in fact more like wrestling with myself: weighing my life, weighing my blog, weighing my choices, and weighing lots of things – lots of weight I was carrying with me. Every once in a blue moon I have this kind of argument with myself. But I am willing to admit it. Not hide it, escape from it, or act as though it doesn't happen. Seeing Joe our teacher for today's class, I was excited, because he seems to say the right thing for our day. I lay on my mat, in the warm Moksha air of 102 degrees, and could've fallen asleep, but after any argument with yourself or others, it is tough to sit still. I focused on the breath, and began to enter my practice. Thank goodness this is a practice.

Even though I spent the first 45 minutes of my morning arguing with myself, my practice was strong, focused, and I noticed something subtle, I was able to listen to myself and toward the tail end, take a break. I was also able to do a transition that was always or has always been a little rough for me. So lots of sweat this morning. Day 28 might be the day that everything turns around, at work, meetings, etc…who knows? I have noticed that through this change of body, mind, and spirit connection, I am being drawn to more positive, outgoing friends, who support, love, and care for me, as much as I do for them. That feels good. My landlady saw me yesterday, and said, "David, I don't know how anyone can't like you? You're really helpful and kind."

I smiled. "Well, Judy, there are probably lots of people out there who don't see me that way, but that's okay, I appreciate that comment, and know that I have a good base of friends, and wonderful daughter who loves me too."

And so Day 28 is over, but my day is just beginning, as I get ready for work, and meetings.

Day 29

Sophie's Choice

Sometimes a person has to go a long distance out their way, to come back a short distance correctly.
– Zoo Story, Edward Albee

Day 29 of 30 straight days of hot yoga at Moksha LA Yoga, it has moved quickly and has been quite the experience for those of you who have been following. I entered class with a new life, the old has slowly evaporated, and during this experience I have found time to breathe lots, and allow the breath to be the guide in the practice. That has made a tremendous difference in my life. I have finally forgiven many people on the road, and by forgiving them, have forgiven myself, and learned a lot about who I am.

Today I lay down on my mat and focused on the breath. As I did this, I followed it down to my hips and back up my spine as I released it. The breath is a great gift and healer. I remembered when Melanie led our class a couple days back and talked about how a bead of sweat is formed and how many different things happen in the body for that to happen. Before Sophie our teacher entered, as I followed the breath, I became aware of the lungs, then the abdominal area, then my organs, the heart, the blood, the millions of cells, and everything in the body being supported by the breath, and everything happening without me getting in the way of it. Thank goodness. I was in awe. And it occurred to me that this body (temple) is given to me as a gift, and one day it will feed the earth, and I have chosen today to nurture it, love it, and appreciate it in my practice.

I have taken Sophie's class many times on this journey and one thing I appreciate is her strength and understanding of the body in the poses. She is a wonderful guide and the practice always feels like an honor. Today she discussed the expression in the pose, that in our practice we sometimes go to what is comfortable, rather than what we don't know. So she offered that up to us in our practice, to explore. In the Tree pose today I couldn't keep my right leg on my thigh; after several attempts, I caught myself looking at everyone else, feeling a sense of looking for approval, or maybe it was wanting to fit in. I was aware of the moment clearly enough, and I was witnessing myself going through it, so I just smiled and moved on.

I felt strong inwardly: bold, and relaxed. As I practice I am happy. I am happy that I followed my intuition here to Moksha, happy that I chose to share my life on the mat with you and not hold back, happy that I continue to learn, happy by letting go, happy about taking care of my temple, happy for all the support from family, friends, and even strangers.

I spent the last several years going way out of my way for everyone, listening to them, taking on their stuff, not listening to myself, feelings of unworthiness, and it feels as if I have finally come home. As a single dad, I know that my daughter is my teacher, I love her, and I am so proud to be her dad, and coach her friends in soccer in the fall. What a blessing this life is.

There is a great juice place next to Moksha called Clover, it is family owned I think, though I'm not sure, and one of the employee's asked me what I will do to celebrate 30 of 30 straight days of yoga. I have no idea, but what I have learned is the moment will reveal itself to me. I will hold in my heart that it will be fun, filled with laughter, joy, some friends, and love.

Day 30

30 for 30

I walked down to Moksha Yoga Los Angeles on my final day. I set out to do 30 straight days of hot yoga, and tonight I finished 30 of 30. I feel happy, I feel strong, and I feel honored. What a thrill to set out on the road, as it weaves in and out, with its roadblocks, twists, and turns. Finally it ends here – all paths start here, and end here. I lay on my mat, closed my eyes, and rested right where I was. I focused on my breath. I followed it down to my hips and out my body, and a word came up, "integrity." Can I be in integrity in each pose? Can I be honest right where I am? Can I be authentic, vulnerable, and alive in the flow? Yes, I can.

Like any practice, we grow, and in this practice I have grown mentally, physically, spiritually, in the past 30 days, I have also discovered something that I feel can only be nurtured through support, love, and care. That quality is vulnerability. Now I look at vulnerability as the opportunity to embrace my imperfections. For example, early on I had moments in some poses where my hips were screaming with sensations, and the mind would rather run away. This happened around day 10 or 11, and I caught myself wanting to hold my face still, as if I was cool in the pose, but inside myself everything was screaming. So in my learning, I would breathe into those places in my being, which were calling for love, the places where the screams were the loudest. As men, we are raised to suck it up, push through pain, hold it all together, be "men," and yet in the practice of yoga, we are called to be with the pose, and breathe into "screams," which goes against the conditioning. It is quite humbling then, to realize that you might not have it all together; you might not know where you are going. But right now, your body's sensations are screaming, calling out for attention, so you leave everything you have learned, and follow the breath into the noise. By embracing the sensations and acknowledging it, not running from it, I open myself up to openness, and embrace the noise.

By doing this, I take an active, alert part in my life – loving myself, by honoring the parts which are scared, hurting, wounded, or shamed. And as I breathe into them they heal, and they heal because I made the choice to nurture, care for, and love those parts. I love the line in Forrest Gump, "I am not a smart man, but I know what love is." Love does not run, does not hide itself, it knows when things are done; it understands, it moves forward, it is patient, kind, and so much more. But when love hears the cries within, it goes to it, and loves it. We are called in our practice to love and accept the parts in each pose that for that day are yearning to be loved.

When I moved to LA to act, I remember my first TV job with an actress who is now known, we were rehearsing the scene and the director said to her, "Now, you see that good-looking man at the bar and you go to him."

I was the only one there on the set, and she said, "Where is the good-looking guy?"

As she made eye contact with me, and I smiled with an uncomfortable look. Inside the voices were going crazy. I raised my hand, and said, "Right here." Silence. Love comes to those places as they show themselves on the mat. I am glad I chose this opportunity to go 30 straight days.

I hope you can go back and read the journey. I have learned so much. I met some wonderful teachers, and it was humbling to practice and learn how to love myself and honor myself. I have spent most of life helping people, and now I have learned the importance of taking care of myself.

Thank you to Emily B and Emily M, Carolina, Joe, Sophie, Katie, Rob, Melanie, and Dalton. To all those who work at Moksha including Ashley in Canada and Jose thank you for spreading the word on the web and To the Moksha family worldwide, and to Moksha LA for winning best yoga studio in LA.

The Choice Point

I finished 30 straight days of hot yoga and the experience was wonderful. I received a challenge from one of my teachers, Emily M, to go for 90 days. I sit with this and it scares me half to death, so I am going for it! 90 straight days of hot yoga, holy cow!

Something that really helped me on my journey so far on the mat and off has really been that of breathing. As a parent in particular, breathing is a wonderful tool, it has allowed me to become a better listener for my daughter, and hear her needs, and as a man has given me permission to feel.

Feeling, as a man in our society, is always or has always been looked down upon, or shunned. But I have realized that it is truly masculine to feel, be vulnerable, and listen. And to take it one more step, we are "beings," and because it is our nature to "to be" here, then breathing is the gateway to feeling. They are interchangeable.

So as I sit here and breath, I announce, "90 days here I come."

Day 31

Going for 90 Days

MOKSHA
mo·ksha
[mohk-shuh] Show IPA
noun Buddhism, Hinduism, Jainism.
freedom from the differentiated, temporal, and mortal world
of ordinary experience.

Well friends, I just finished 30 straight days of hot yoga at
Moksha Yoga Los Angeles, and just when I thought it was over,
life has invited me to go further, so I am going for 90 straight
days. I love the community of Moksha Los Angeles and Moksha,
it is a powerful, green, sustainable community of yogis.

In my first 30 days I learned a lot about breath, alignment,
grace, strength, and vulnerability. As I lay on my mat today, I
needed it, I had just spent six hours planting and mulching at my
daughter's new school, and my arms, legs where sore. And when
I showed up to practice yoga, I set my intention to explore the
sore.

Katie guided us through a wonderful practice of Yang/Yin. It
felt good to stretch out. I noticed in my practice that when I am
sore, how easy it is to contract. So as I became aware of the
contraction, I allowed myself to breathe with it and it helped with
expanding my poses. As I expanded, it felt as though my arms
were releasing the soreness and it helped me relax. As I relaxed
into it, I discovered the wonder of the breath again, observing
how it moved through the stuck parts of the body. As the breath
expanded through the stuck parts, the breath became deeper,
fuller, and I felt Zen-like.

There is a wonderful story of an older Zen master who was

challenged by a younger warrior. The older Zen masters students explained how rough, and strong the younger warrior was and how frightened they were that their teacher would be harmed. So the older Zen master went outside and stood six feet away from the young warrior. The young warrior, screamed at him, yelled profanities, spat on him, called him names, called his family names, and finally after several hours quit and walked away. When the older Zen master appeared back inside, his students were amazed. "Master how come you did nothing, the young warrior belittled you, called you names, spat on you, and you did nothing."

The master explained, "When someone gives you a gift and you do not take it, whose gift does it belong to?"

They thought about it. "The one who gave it."

The master said, "Yes."

In yoga we are given many gifts on our mat, some are loud sensations, loud voices, and loud drama, and yet we have a choice to take the gift and play into the drama of it or not. It's up to you. By not contracting I was taking the gift, and the gift was teaching me to expand, not contract. Yes, I was sore today, yes, it's easy to give in, but the gift was to open. It is easy to listen to the mind and give up, play small, but the opportunity is to breathe and go into it. The gift is to shine from the inside out. We are here to liberate ourselves and be free. Are you in?

Detox, Cleanse, and Weight Loss

As I walked to Moksha Yoga LA on day 32 of 90 straight days of hot yoga, I contemplated a dream with a friend. The dream offered me insight into my newfound stability, growth, and expression. I like entering the Moksha studio, it is a representation of walking into a temple. The sign asks us to maintain silence in the room. As I contemplated my journey on the mat I was aware of my toes, and then I became aware of the space between them, and as this happened, my breath deepened. I began to become aware of the space between my fingers, organs, the space outside of me, and inside, and realized this breath is always filling the space. It reminds me of water as it fills ever space and moves around things with ease and grace.

Our teacher Joe emphasized the importance of the breath, gravity, and how the breath moves without force. The breath comes into our bodies and exhales. "Let gravity help your pose, use it." As I practiced I had a flash of questions. How many times do I allow my breath to be? Or allow gravity to ground me? Or Allow life to flow now? Well as I continue to practice Moksha Yoga, I am finding out.

Some poses flow with grace, and others are inhibited by my mind, but when I acknowledge the breath and trust the breath in the pose, it takes me to a more open space inside and then the expression is very dynamic and purposeful. It is funny, I just looked up "PURR" and it is defined as "To signify or express by purring." So your purpose in life is your self-expression. Awesome. And your self-expression allows you to purr like a cat with contentment. So life is purpose, every moment offering self-expression and contentment in the expression.

I have tried many practices of detoxifying – cleansing – and so far this practice offers a whole being experience. Meaning that it has helped build compassion for others, unifying the body, mind, and spirit, and me, while detoxifying and cleansing the system as well and it only takes 60–75 minutes a day. I have lost nine pounds, and my diet has merged into a healthy based way of being in the world. I feel good, and I am starting to notice difference in the mental realm (more peace of mind), and in the physical realm (I am becoming stronger, focused, and purposeful), and finally in the spiritual realm (I am allowing the breath to guide the practice which allows me to honor my temple). Heaven on earth is the unification of body, mind, and spirit. Onward to day 33…

Day 33 of 90

Noticing

As I approached day 33 of 90 straight days of Moksha Yoga LA I was tired. I entered the studio at 7:30 am, lay on my mat and closed my eyes. Feeling the floor below me and letting gravity pull me down, I focused on the breath. It was here I noticed the shift from feeling tired to feeling a little invigorated. The invigoration was the awareness of commitment. Here I am committing to 90 straight days of hot yoga, and like any and all commitments whether with ourselves, another person, company, health, a dream and so forth, we have our ebb and flow. The movement of life – some days flow and others seem a little bumpy, but we show up, or "should" because those are prisons, and we commit ourselves not out of obligation, but because we can. The commitment comes from our willingness to show up fully. And showing up fully might be going through things; so we notice those spaces within us that don't want to be here, that don't want to be with whatever is happening now within us.

Today in practice, Sophie brought up this concept of "noticing." So, for example, we had our eyes closed standing up and I felt wobbly, and Sophie asked us to just notice how we were feeling now. It was quite powerful, because if I am feeling upset, and I notice it, then I think, and I don't want to feel upset, so try to change it. By trying to change it, it makes it worse. By noticing the upset and committing fully with it, it passes through. But if I notice it and then play into the drama of it, then that is a different feeling. This is what I mean, as I move where I am and feel the upset and just notice it, the feeling falls away on its own, but, on the other hand, if I notice frustration and then decide that this feeling is who I am, then I play out the drama of frustration, "I am always frustrated." Do you see? I am not always frustrated it is the energy of frustration passing through. So Moksha practice is teaching me to liberate myself by noticing the feeling without changing it or identifying with it, and accepting it now, and then allowing it to pass through. That is quite different from what we are taught.

This is wonderful news. We live in a society that is always wanting to change us, fix us, judge us, criticize us, because that is how we are with ourselves, denying the feeling because we don't want it. Have you ever been around people that the moment you mention you are feeling bad, they jump on it, want to fix it, change you, and all the rest of it, or worse still love it and want to hold you down. Yoga is about the experience, and each experience is leading us to the next, but our job is to be fully committed to it. For each pose is bringing us into the next, and each pose is offering us a chance to experience our feelings, sensations, bodies, and thoughts as they are, in the hopes of liberating our identities from them.

Day 34 of 90

Mona Lisa…Ending Perfection

I entered day 34 of 90 straight days of hot yoga at Moksha Yoga Los Angeles with a sense of renewed vigor for my practice. Last night I practiced and found some new understanding in my practice, and some strength. Our teacher Carolina explained the story of Warrior poses and where they came from and their meaning. After hearing the story I felt such purpose in my Warrior poses and strength, so entering morning class today, I felt renewed. I lay on the mat, closed my eyes, and let gravity pull me down, and let my breath rise and fall.

As the breath was falling I had an image of the Mona Lisa painting, and then other images of statues and artwork. What occurred to me was that every good work of art starts with an empty canvas or a block of clay, and the artist gets an inspired idea of what it may look like and begins to paint and build from there. Yet each stroke of paint is adding to the beauty of the work. So within the so-called perfection of a painting or statue is the imperfection of it all. The imperfection allows the so-called perfect art to shine. Essentially, all art is beautiful because it embraces the imperfection, just as yoga practice does. Yoga encourages you to fall, laugh, be imperfect, and get up and try again.

As our teacher Lisa started practice I felt imperfect in every pose, and I started chuckling to myself. I dropped out a few times and came back into it smiling. Lisa was wonderful and focused us on alignment and maintaining the poses for extended periods with great care and gentleness. Helping us find the grace of the breath in each pose. By falling, we learn to get up, and then we learn from the fall. Yoga is like great art, each of us has an idea of what it may look or feel like, or we may have read some yoga magazine forgetting the models took five hours to get the pose right before they took the shot and published it, or we have seen masters hold poses or do them with ease, forgetting that for years and years they were moving through their own imperfection to perfect the moment.

Life is a balance between imperfect and perfect. I have noticed that the majority of my practice is imperfect, falling, and regrouping. Years ago this would have driven me up the wall. Because I wanted perfection in my life, I wanted life to be ideal, and felt people should know better, but frankly we learn that life is all about embracing this – this as it is. Observing it, experiencing it, and then allowing the next pose or moment in life to flow. So be imperfect and embrace it.

I used to take classes where the teachers would ask students to come in front of class because they thought their practice was incredible. Then the mind says, "Well, that is what I am going for" or "Wow, I can never do that." Cut to now, and I realize that life is not about comparing, competing, but celebrating each other. Celebrating our life as a yoga community through consciously making choices in our practice to embrace the fall, the imperfect, each other, and say, "Yes I can." Behind our imperfection is perfection glowing, shining, and cheering us on. We are all here on purpose and each of us makes a difference to someone and this planet.

Day 35 of 90

"Karma, Sweat, and Music"

I was excited to enter the studio today for day number 35 of 90 straight days of hot yoga at Moksha Yoga LA. Today's class had live music by Dalton and he rocked it. It was a 75-minute class with teacher Joe and Dalton; it was wonderful. Such a vibrant community of people practicing to live music, wonderful guidance by Joe, and lots and lots of sweat. Before class I lay on my mat and took in my day. I was filled with much gratitude for it. I have received such kind letters of support from people on this journey of 90 days, so thank you. I love the support.

In class Joe our teacher talked about the importance of giving, the importance of the breath, and the importance of focus in our practice, allowing us to become aware of our breath and the rise and fall in each pose. Also, Joe talked about giving and getting. What we give we get. It reminds me of karma, which means "comeback." You judge and you will be judged, you criticize and you will be criticized, you love and you will be loved, you control and you will be controlled. The funny thing about karma (action) is you can't run from it, you have to deal with it now. In our practice as we give ourselves kindness, gentleness, and compassion, then the pose gives us back kindness, gentleness, and compassion. Forgiveness always erases karmic actions that hurt others and releases us as well from the debt. Because when we hurt others, we are hurting ourselves. But the forgiveness has to be sincere and from the heart. Just like our practice on the mat. We show up humbled, and sincere, and allow our breath to guide us in and out of the pose. I noticed something very funny tonight. I learned somewhere and it doesn't matter where, that when you work, you should look serious. So I caught myself breathing into a pose with a serious look and started giggling. "Good grief!"

and how quickly the practice can humble us. How quickly we can be humbled by pride, by feeling right all the time, or by taking life too serious.

Life is experience, and experience on the mat is a great teacher. It teaches us as Joe said, "How to breathe with the body on and off the mat." We learn the importance of breathing in each pose, the importance of breathing in life, and the importance of coming from our hearts in a sincere way. Karma strikes when we least expect it, you may have harmed another life through lies, deceit, hate, unkindness, and cheating, and think you got away with it. But nature teaches us, none us get away with it; nature balances things out. When others are unkind to us, observe how it feels, breathe a couple of times, and respond from a different place. Sometimes it's best to just walk away, and say nothing. And send these people good thoughts. Because people who treat you unkindly are probably working through hurt, and what looks like unkindness is a call for love. Most people who are hurting inside are calling out for love. Life is not personal, the meaning we put on life makes it personal. So be gentle with your story, be gentle with yourself, and be gentle with people. Everyone is doing their best. At the end of your day, ask yourself, "How much did I love today? Did I love as much as I could? Did I hold back?" Yoga gives us the opportunity to express fully our love from the inside out.

Give love, give kindness, and give compassion.

Day 36 of 90

Gravity and Breath

I walked into day 36 of 90 straight days of hot yoga at Moksha Yoga LA with an intention to extend. I lay on my mat, closed my eyes and focused on my breath. As I lay there resting in my breath, I became aware of my legs extending, my arms extending at my side, and the breath extending. I felt gravity pulling me down on my mat, and the space of the room around me.

Dalton our teacher entered and we focused on the breath, and allowing it to bring us deeper into the poses. How wonderful, that when you rest in the breath, it takes you into each pose gently. What really helped me out was last week when our teacher Joe mentioned gravity, and letting gravity pull you down. So today when I was in my poses I focused on gravity pulling me down and then allowing the breath to take over. What was interesting was how much resisting I was doing in the poses, but once I allowed gravity to work and my breath to work in each one, it took me in deeper, along with the guidance of Dalton and his instruction. He mentioned to us in the class, "I know this burns your legs holding it for a couple of breaths." It was burning but by staying focused on the earth pulling me down and my breathing, it helped me stay deeper and allowed me to extend with stronger purpose. Also I noticed that I was able to begin to feel the rotation of the body in different poses as well. Going with the pose, with the flow, sounds easy, but it can be hard. And today I found the flow and began flowing into the poses. Having a foundation really makes a huge difference and these past 36 days have been helping me build a healthy foundation. My foundation is built with gentleness, compassion, and giggles. I am not taking myself so seriously and that is making a whole lot of difference.

I hope this journey is helping you as well and I thank you for your continued support. As I move into day 37 I am reminded that life is happening now, the rest is all speculation. So enjoy yourself here and be open to the possibilities life presents. I remember speaking at Unity Burbank one time, and as my daughter and I left in the car, she said, "Dad, I know what you do?"

I said, "What?"

She smiled and said, "My dad loves people."

That can be difficult sometimes when we are moving through things off our mat and on. I have moved through many situations and what I am learning is, no matter what, to know that "I am okay now."

Day 37 of 90

What is My Motivation?

I walked into day 37 of 90 straight days of hot yoga at Moksha Yoga LA with a thought moving in my awareness. "What is my motivation?" As I continue to practice on my yoga mat, I am noticing the benefits off it as well, including patience, and mindfulness. An example of this was last night. I was about to say something to someone and stopped, then the questions came, "What is my motivation here? Is this the right time to share this? Will these words harm or help the conversation?" I was shocked. At the end of the night I spoke with clarity and love. So I felt like bringing this mindfulness practice to my mat today. As I lay on it I felt it on my back, and also the breath in my body, the space between my toes, the space between my legs, I felt the heaviness of the body, and felt the silence in the room and I asked, "What is my motivation in today's practice?" The answer, "Mindfulness."

Our teacher Sophie entered the room, and asked us to engage the breath and let the breath be active in the pose. To stay in the breath as we moved. My practice was what it was today. As I was mindful in the practice I was able to feel different places in the body and able to really feel how different body parts are engaged and active in each pose. I was mindful of my tired states, my active states, my states where the mind wanted to come in, and when mind came in how I felt, and then would remind myself to breathe again. I notice when my mind comes in and starts thinking, I am probably not breathing. So today was a dance of consciousness, allowing mindfulness, breath, to adjust and move the body.

It is funny how quickly our inner guide responds with quick, clear answers. I smiled again. When I breathe and have no thoughts hindering me in the pose, I notice my practice to be fluid and really flow, but when the mind comes in, well the toppling tree falls over and I feel constricted, and resistance takes over. Today's practice was a wonderful learning curve for me, to stay mindful in my practice and smile.

Day 38 of 90

IS?

As I entered day 38 of 90 straight days of hot yoga at Moksha Yoga LA I was a little sluggish but excited for my practice. I lay briefly on my mat this morning and contemplated the warmth of the room and the word "IS" entered my mind. I love yoga. I love it because every day on my mat there is something to be with, explore, and most importantly breathe with as well. As I sat with the word "IS," some words came forward to join it, "inner strength" and "inner spirit." I have heard the "ISness of life," or "be with what is," and I have had a difficult time with the latter. But being with the sense that "IS" can be looked at as "inner spirit" really relaxed my body and mind. When I am completely present in my breath I am really in my inner spirit of each pose, or inner strength. Spirit to me is strength, so there is no difference for me.

Today teacher Joe really focused us on the inner guide and listening to the source within, reminding us of the breath within and staying connected to the inner guide, listening to it, and checking in to see if we need to take breaks, and staying grounded in the earth and letting gravity work. As I have brought up on a number of writings, I love this idea of gravity pulling you down and grounding your poses. Today's practice offered me freedom, focus and inner strength. It is very powerful, because now I see how the mind wants to pull me away from my authentic, innate inward power. So in my poses I enjoyed the presence a lot more and watched how weak the mind is. Now I know why the present moment is a gift, it is offering us so much. Eckhart Tolle is right about "The Power of Now." There is great power here.

That said, it is quite challenging to work with the process of coming here now, so be gentle, be kind to yourself in your discovery. We all have our moments. I feel as if today's practice really gave me a point to come back to when the mind wanders away as it sometimes does. I simply bring my attention to "I.S." the inner spirit dwelling now and dwelling in all of us, and when I connect with it, life becomes full of riches and great wealth.

Day 39 of 90

Yin and The Plant

I moved into day 39 of 90 straight days of hot yoga at Moksha Yoga with a gentle practice called Yin. I was looking forward to this with a busy week approaching. Yin is a practice that has long holds, and helps in restoring the body with longer stretches and breathing. I like to do this at least twice a week. It helps me with clarity and peace of mind. It has been beneficial in many phases of my life, and I am grateful for Yin.

Teacher Sophie led our class; she is wonderfully insightful, and full of wonderful teachings, and humor. I like her style, and enjoy how she meets you right where you are. As a case in point, I was in a pose and she helped me into it, talked with me about it, and then supported me in it. When we worked the second side, she made me aware of the other side and how much more open it was. As people, we always feel better when others meet us right where we are. I also enjoy her music. At the end of class I was reminded of a story.

There was a plant that was in a small pot. In the small pot it felt tight, constricted, and couldn't grow. Then one day, it was taken out of the small pot and placed into a bigger pot. Now the plant felt so much more space it didn't know what to do. There was so much space it began to panic; it was not used to so much space. But as it began to stretch out its roots, it felt freedom, and aliveness. The plant felt the rays of the sun, the breeze, and the gentle rain. It began to enjoy it all. It began to enjoy its newfound freedom.

As I am practicing every day in hot yoga, I am starting to understand my practice, and embrace a new sense of whom I am. It has been a very long time coming. But I am starting to feel strong, more vibrant, and alive. Today felt good coming into a community like Moksha in Los Angeles. It felt good to sit and talk with people and laugh before practice. These past 39 days have been quite insightful, inspiring, challenging, and humorous. Congratulations Teacher Joe on your engagement.

Day 40 of 90

The Big 4-0

Today marks number 40 of 90 straight days of hot yoga at Moksha Yoga and it also marks opportunity. As I entered my 40th day, I also entered a day that has many different options. We all make plans and then those plans shift and we have to go with the flow. I have learned and continue to learn to fly with it. Be with it. And most importantly, as I am with it, whatever it is. I am called to be gentle, kind, and compassionate with myself, because if I am not gentle, kind, and compassionate with myself, well then I will expect you to give me that, because I don't give myself it, and then I become powerless. But I am here to liberate myself, not be powerless.

I lay on my mat and decided to practice with the tip of my tongue on the roof of my mouth, which is wonderful and very helpful with keeping me calm and relaxed in the poses. It really helps with calming the mind. I use this when I meditate and I decided to test it out today. It also helped with relaxing my face and allowing me to breathe deeply.

Our teacher today was Lisa who brought up something early on, which I loved, "Meet yourself on your mat," which really added to my day. We spend so much time meeting others where they are that we forget to meet ourselves right where we are. Lisa was wonderful with helping us to align in the pose, with being gentle, and guiding us with kind reminders. It helped me see that we are so kind, helpful, and compassionate with others, that it reminded me to speak to myself that way. You and I are very important to lots of people. Now I might not see that all the time, but I am pretty sure my five-year-old daughter sees me that way. Therefore, I am an important example to my daughter on how I treat myself. I did this challenge because as a dad, my daughter is watching my actions not my words. If I am kind, gentle, and compassionate as things are unfolding then she will see the importance of loving yourself, and caring for yourself, and knowing that our words matter, that we matter.

So I am an example for a future leader, contributor, and lover to this planet, who is always watching me. I love sharing this story, and as a teacher myself, sometimes it is a great reminder of true teaching: A mom brought her son to see Gandhi and asked him to tell her son to get off sugar.

Gandhi replied, "Come back in 30 days." So 30 days later she came back, and Gandhi saw her son and said, "Get off sugar."

The mom inquired, "Why did it take you 30 days?"

He smiled, and replied, "Because I had to get off it first."

I can't tell my daughter to be kind, share, have compassion, forgive, love, if in fact I don't walk that way myself. I can only tell her what I know, my experience. It starts with me. I must be kind, compassionate, and gentle with me. The lesson for me as a parent, single dad, friend, son, teacher, student, speaker, counselor, facilitator, writer, blogger, and all the parts I play in between, is speak what you live. If we don't know the answer, then we don't know. But we will learn. In yoga when I fall, I fall, and then I get up and learn. Yoga is life and life is happening here, right here, so let's practice kindness for each other, and only speak what we know for ourselves to be true.

Day 41 of 90

Granted

I walked into day 41 of 90 straight days of hot yoga at Moksha Yoga LA and placed my mat down. Lying down in the room, and following my breath, I focused on the abundance of breath that is breathing me now, and how much I take my breath for granted, how much I take this life for granted, and even how others have taken me for granted, or I have taken others for granted. So I was led on my mat by the word "granted." It sounds funny in a yoga class, to be contemplating the word "granted." What is granted? Well in the dictionary, granted is to acknowledge, recognize or make known.

In my 41 days of liberation so far on the mat, I spent pretty much most of practice acknowledging my breath, acknowledging who I am, acknowledging my path, acknowledging and recognizing what is here, and understanding what I used to take for granted in my life. So I decided to feel thankful for the practice today and continued to rest in gentleness with myself. It is a blessing to be practicing, it is a blessing to have a body that works, a blessing to walk, and do yoga, and it is a blessing to acknowledge my breath, which breathes me without judgment. My breath never judges me, or others. It breathes everyone equally and is opportunistic and inspiring.

Today teacher Lisa led us in what she calls, "The symphony of the body." Our practice explored the breath, space, and alignment of each pose. I found and discovered some better alignment in Tree pose and found easier ways to be in it. I never realized how hard I could make things, but as I followed the breath and relaxed into it, the pose happened without me doing anything, just going with the flow. This week I had plans to get away with my daughter but life came in and changed the plans.

So without questioning it, I went with it and moved on. It was a good lesson on moving with life. It can be difficult to move when we have expectations, or others let us down, but we are called in every aspect of our life to keep moving with it, move with the pose on the mat, move with life, move with grace, and move with breath.

Lisa spent time demonstrating the pose for some people that were new to the practice and it was great to watch her. I was able to learn again and see where my placement was and I did not take it for granted. Life is granted to us, and because it is granted to us, we are called to discover love, discover the Divine within, and rid ourselves of fear. The call is always to come inward. So stay in your temple and look out onto the world. Let us not take anything for granted, not even each other. This life is unfolding for us here and never lets us down. Life is our friend, and our breath is our good buddy.

Day 42 of 90

Dream Big

Day 42 of 90 straight days of hot yoga at Moksha Yoga LA and in yesterday's post I talked about the idea of "granted" and today our teacher was Grant, funny, but an answered prayer. Grant really enforced again, the power of the breath, and really reminded our class today of the moments we stop breathing. I notice in my life off the mat that I stop breathing when I forget to allow life to unfold. Grant has tremendous strength both inwardly and outwardly. It was wonderful to experience his teaching and I feel blessed for the opportunity.

In flow I have been having trouble with a certain pose. I discovered with the help from Grant, by inhaling into the pose it pulls the pressure off my lower back and lets me into it in the correct way. I will tell you right now, "hallelujah." I have been really working with this and today it clicked into place. I felt such power and inner strength in the pose as well. That same type of breath really helped in sustaining my other poses, and I am beginning to experience the breath and pose as one movement.

Before today I didn't realize that they appeared separate to my practice. Today they became one. I caught myself in the mirror and saw inner and outer strength. What I love is that by being gentle, kind, and patient with myself, and not pushing it, I have slowly developed a strong foundation that I can come to. That is very important to me.

In my life, when things fell apart, I didn't have a healthy foundation to go to. True I had meditation, prayer and affirmations, but when things fell completely apart, I fell over and would eat badly, punish and judge myself, and even experience much shame. What does that mean? It means that when life offered me a right hook, I caved in and fell down, and I didn't want to get up. I would give up on myself. I felt worthless, and low.

So now I am noticing that by doing yoga every day, I am developing a healthy way to handle life and its challenges. I am breathing with things, even when the answer doesn't come. I am starting to work with life, not against it. I understand that "this will pass" and if it does come back, it isn't as strong as the first time.

As I write this I can only think of each of you and how we inspire each other. Truly thank you for allowing me the opportunity to share and grow before you. I hope my journey can inspire you and allow you to see that as you pursue your dreams there are challenges, but if you are patient, kind, and gentle with yourself in the process of it, that life will offer you support and love.

Day 43 of 90

Follow the Silly

Day 43 of 90 straight days of hot yoga at Moksha Yoga LA, with the practice of Yang/Yin. I entered the studio and lay down on the mat, closed my eyes and relaxed, allowing gravity to pull me down. My life off the mat is starting to take shape, move and expand. It has been a long road and every step has been earned, and learned. We are always learning to relax into the present and listen and keep moving. The mind disagrees with this and holds on to everything.

Rob our teacher is really quite fun. He is a paradox as a teacher. I am a good listener, and Rob's voice is calm, soft, and strong, yet our practice can be quite vigorous with lots of flow. But I love how much he understands both the Yang/Yin of our practice and I learned a lot about my body as well. I have eased off on the flow classes for three days to focus on my foundation and it helped a lot in today's flow, I was strong and active, and really felt the surrender into the breath. I heard the "SHHHHH" of the breath again and kept the tip of the tongue on the roof of the mouth. All of which allows the mind to calm and it really activates the AB area, and helps center me.

There was a point in my practice where I felt my heart was smiling for the very first time in a long time. Time heals and so does forgiveness. Together they have really healed an interesting stage of my life, all of which has opened me up to vulnerability and a deeper connection to the Divine, my daughter, and myself.

My daughter and I were taking a long walk last night, she was talking about something and I asked, "How did that feel?"

She said, "It made me feel silly."

"Okay, does silly feel good?"

She said, "Dad, silly feels silly."

So I said, "Follow the silly feeling, but remember always to feel what you feel, because that matters."

We continued to walk, and about five minutes after our conversation, my daughter said, "Dad, I love you so much."

"I love you too."

Day 44 of 90

Courtship and Cupid

Well day 44 of 90 straight days of hot yoga at Moksha Yoga LA, finds me in the middle of long courtship, a very long courtship. As I lay on my mat, closed my eyes and focused on my breath, two strange questions came up, "Who would I be without my breath?" and "Who would I be without my thoughts?" And so my journey started today from there. The funny thing was the answers. "Dead," was the answer to the first question And the answer to the second was "I would soar!" As I felt the answer in my body, the soaring felt wonderful, and I glimpsed myself without a thought: such freedom too!

Emily B our teacher entered the womb (studio), and brought up in Moksha class today the idea of focusing on what she called, "Cupid," the marriage of mind and breath in the practice. She asked us to "notice" ourselves in each pose. Simply notice how we are being in each pose, while marrying the mind and breath together. It was then I realized that I have been in a courtship for many years, and today my breath, whom I call Grace, met her man (Men-tal). In today's practice their courtship began. For the first time they noticed each other and they liked what they saw. Grace appreciated the Men-tal's excitement to go and take the adventure, and in turn, the Men-tal appreciated Grace with her strength, patience, and compassion. Together they merged in a union in each pose. When the Men-tal wanted to push, Grace brought her breath in and balanced the pose. It was a wonderful dance of breath and mind working together with the body.

I noticed how much stronger I have become in each pose, and in some of the others I have noticed how quickly I wanted to run. But I was able to use Emily's tool of noticing the pose itself and then my breath helped balance me into it, with grace. Practice today had slower movements into the poses and I loved it. I was able to notice places that I wanted to simply push through and not rest in. It was also helpful to have the mind and breath work together. I realize this is practice and so it feels good to see movement and growth and places to go into. The courtship continues...

Day 45 of 90

Nonviolence

It is day 45 of 90 straight days of hot yoga at Moksha Yoga LA and as I entered the halfway point of this adventure into vulnerability, compassion, and the life within, I realized that our culture, which means cult, spends much time defending the outer; and so when I mention nonviolence I am sure the focus outside goes to guns, wars, and all the rest of it.

But in this book we are going to focus on the inward life. When it's quiet and you are alone listening to yourself, are you beating yourself up, judging, criticizing, and shaming yourself, or even thinking about regrets and resentments? My own discovery on the mat has been one of going into the inner war and bringing peace to it. What would my life look like, feel like, and be like? Without inner violence I can walk a nonviolent life inside myself. The second half of this journey is to walk in nonviolence against myself.

Our teacher Carolina introduced the idea of taking our time with the practice, giving ourselves breaks, and breathing with the poses. This goes along the lines of my intention today in class, to bring nonviolence to my pose. So I met each one with nonviolence and where I started to beat myself up, no worries, as I brought more breath into the pose to relax the Yang, and bring more love in. The breath is love. Every time you breathe, you love yourself. When you think endlessly, you will notice the breath stops, and then you become shallow in your breath and in your life. I love breathing, it is a simple act of love for myself.

Today I added to my new way of being in life as a nonviolent yogi, by going next door to Cover Juice, and I am glad I did. Most students after class go to Clover and get a juice. I have decided to eat healthily by adding a juice to my day. Clover is a wonderful place filled with employees who are friendly and outgoing. My daughter chose me a juice called the Black Chia. Filled with agave, water, and chia, it was delicious and really helped me after practice today. So if you get a chance to do Moksha, go next door and try a juice. I am excited now to go to Clover and add it to my nonviolent inner lifestyle. I love taking care of myself and health is a huge factor, it tells the heart you care.

Day 46 of 90

Yin and the Taste of Mint

I walked into day 46 of 90 straight days of hot yoga at Moksha Yoga LA after a long day of soccer meetings downtown. I decided to get a juice at Clover Juice next door before my practice. My energy was low and so I bought a drink called CLEAN GREEN, simply because it said, "energize." Wow it was a wonderful pick me up and my breath smelled fantastic. It also has Chlorophyll, Peppermint Oil, and H2O. Within a few minutes I was reignited to practice. I love juice where the ingredients are simple and that they use locally grown stuff. CLEAN GREEN is wonderful to take before any workout.

I entered the studio for a Yin practice. Our teacher Emily B is a wonderfully insightful, and a very intuitive teacher. I love her Yin class. We go, we let go, and we go deep into the tissues. I was able to see in my practice today how quickly the mind wants to come in and create a story, and the story has nothing to do with what is actually happening. I was also able to see in the stillness how beautiful I am.

Now for me to say that has taken some time. Do I realize in my life that some people might not see that in me? Yes. Do I also know there are people who see that same beauty in me? Yes. But I also realize that can change with people, and what matters is that I see it, and feel it. Because, as I discovered in my practice, the mind will trick you into listening to its stories and it can be subtle as well. In today's practice I felt very deep, still, and rested in each pose. I love that.

I am realizing that by having a healthy diet, by taking care of my health, loving myself right where I am, and not pushing for more, that I rest in gratefulness and feel so much gratitude without looking for it. I realize it is here, right here. That the beauty I saw in the stillness of myself is everywhere. I bring that up because sometimes I have to write a list of things I am grateful for when I forget. So health leads to wealth. I am now moving towards the unity of mind, body, and spirit, and resting in the present moment more with each practice. The "present" is the gift we give to each other.

Day 47 of 90

How Am I Feeling Now?

Day 47 of 90 straight days of hot yoga at Moksha Yoga LA, and before practice I noticed something that seem to shift my life. I noticed that I was feeling a little down. I can't really explain why, but it lasted for a few minutes, until this question arose, "How am I feeling now?" The answer was, "Low." So I asked myself, "What is this low feeling from?" The answer came back, "Focusing on what you don't want." So I asked, "Can I change this feeling?" and I started to focus on what I wanted. As I did this, my feelings began to rise up. I felt lighter, thankful, and alive. In one fell swoop the great law of love came in. We are here to love. Love is being and being is feeling. As you are present you are feeling fully the great love, the big love, the Divine. From this place you have a choice, to love or fear.

So for my practice today I decided to lie down on my mat, and feel the mat below, feel my body, feel the breath, and then ask, "How am I feeling now?" The answer was "Relaxed." I sank into my mat with my eyes closed and felt empowered.

A good example for me is this path I am on, writing on my 90 straight days of hot yoga; now let's say you don't like this, and I hear you. And let's say after I hear you, I need to be liked, so if you don't like it, then I feel let down, unworthy, lost, because I cared more about how you feel than how I feel. Now I can ask myself, "How am I feeling now?" The answer is "Disempowered." Now I am honest with myself, and not negating the feeling. So now I ask, "Can I change this feeling?" The answer is "Yes." Now I am empowered again, I have a choice.

Our teacher Charis entered the class with a wonderful style of intelligence, strength, and love. She guided us through the practice, with style, and wonderful music. She was attentive and spent time helping us when we needed it. Now in today's class I caught myself wobbling in a pose, which is fine, but my wobbling was coming from my focus on a student in front of me who was wobbling. I checked in and asked myself, "How am I feeling now?" The answer was "Unfocused" I asked, "Can I change this feeling?" The answer was "Yes." I went inside and allowed my breath to guide my practice and my attention went from outside to inside. I stopped wobbling. Our feelings are wonderful indicators of what we are focusing on, and when we change them, we empower ourselves. We empower our lives. So when you find yourself in a feeling of negativity, ask yourself, "How am I feeling now?" And then ask, "Can I change this feeling?" See where it takes you! Love you. Tomorrow I start a three day cleanse with Clover…I will share my thoughts.

Day 48 of 90

Hello Down Dog

Day 48 of 90 straight days of hot yoga at Moksha LA, and I was reminded today of the simplicity of the word "Hello." When was the last time you simply just sat next to someone and said, "Hello"? Instead we are always concerned and ask, "How is your day going?" or "What do you do for a living?" or "How are you doing?" In yoga we meet every pose with "Hello," then we are silent with it and rest in the gift it is giving us. The poses don't change, our interpretations of them changes. Have you ever sat with someone, and said, "Hello," and then just sat there in the silence, resting in your own insecurity with space, with the silence, without wanting to add something or change them, and just enjoying the space?

Today in class our teacher Joe brought forth some gems, including that the breath will get you through anything in life. It is strong and amazing. Yoga reminds me a beautiful rose, and as the rose is growing we don't yell at the rose to grow faster, change, be different, or be what we want it to be. No, in fact we accept it – we accept that the rose is growing and we are patient with it.

So how come when we are growing and moving through things, we yell at ourselves, try to push through it, change it, be different, why is a rose different from who we are? The same is true about the word, "Hello." Why does it matter what someone does for a living? Why does it matter if they are having a good day or bad day? Does that change how we are with them? If they say they are famous, am I different with them? If they say they are homeless am I different with them? If they say they are having a difficult day, or great day, does that change me? When we say, "Hello" we are really saying, "Love." And love meets itself right where it is, and accepts itself here, just like yoga practice. There is nothing to change, or fix. "Hello Warrior pose" or "Hello Down dog." Then with our breath the adjustments happen in their own time. We are, each of us, like a beautiful rose growing in our own time under the sun.

Final note, I started a three-day juice cleanse today with the help of Clover Juice. I am only seven hours into it. I feel great, I am drinking lots of water, and the juice so far is fantastic. I am about to drink an afternoon snack of carrot, apple, and ginger. It is bright orange and vibrant. I started this juice fast because I read that our bodies hold 5–10 pounds of toxins in our intestines, and I just about fell off my chair. I also love that when I awoke and drank a juice called Rev'd Up it packed a power punch and really woke me up. It lasted longer than the coffee I normally drink.

Day 49 of 90

You Have the Power

Day 49 of 90 days straight of hot yoga at Moksha Yoga LA and I was up early. I entered practice today with teacher Joe and felt tired. Today's class was at 6 am but my day is busy. So I lay down on my mat, closed my eyes and just relaxed into the warmth of the room. As we started practice I noticed some nice things starting to blossom in my practice. I am focused, gentle with myself, and kind. My practice is starting to align in certain poses, while in others it finds its way. I am good with that. The breath is a wonderful tool off my mat as well. As things come up, I am able to breathe and relax into clarity.

These past 49 days have allowed be to grow in other areas as well. I am on day two of a juice cleanse I thought I would try at Clover Juice. Last night was a little difficult my head was pounding from no caffeine. But that is normal. This morning I feel great and craving the juice and water. I will have to say that this fast is very well put together. I have had no cravings and I am drinking a juice about every two hours. And I love that if I have any questions, I can always ask. My body feels great from yoga and juicing.

I am also blossoming as a parent. My daughter and I are having blast. I have been teaching her how to listen to her feelings and trust them. I can do that now, because I am doing it myself. Each of our lives is important, and it is important that we feel our feelings, be in our bodies, and experience life now. I know this sounds simple, but sometimes it is very difficult to stand here and express what you are feeling to someone. Life never stops, life doesn't hold on, it keeps moving, and as we empty our minds of the past, and dwell in the present, we begin to see that we really do have a choice now, to be happy or not.

Happiness doesn't depend on something, or someone to be itself. It is a choice. We can choose to be negative, but really being negative is an easy choice, a lazy choice, and anyone can do that. What is difficult is accepting and choosing to be positive. Forgiveness, love, grace, humility, and compassion take practice. They take inner strength. Life is a practice, practicing to love.

"How are you being?" Everything you are being right now is a choice. Be happy, be sad, be whatever, but it all starts here, with you. No one can make you do, feel anything – NO ONE. You have the power to choose.

Day 50 of 90

The Big 5-0

Day 50 of 90 straight days of hot yoga at Moksha Yoga LA and I arrived to hear two people singing and playing a guitar in the lobby. Quite fun. I am finishing my 50th straight day of hot yoga and love that after class I received a text message from a woman on the east coast who was inspired by my journey, and has enrolled in a yoga class to start her journey. Yoga inspires.

Tonight I lay on my mat and dove into my breath. Teacher Joe was on fire with his wisdom and guiding us through our practice. At one point he offered us an invitation, to do the last half of practice with our eyes closed. Those who have been reading this journey know that I spent a class early on with my eyes closed, but this time I noticed something. Joe always mentions the intuitive breath, and tonight I noticed the intuitive breath within my own temple. With my eyes closed I felt the breath within my body and felt it align my shoulder blades and my spine, and like a gentle massage, open my heart up. Joe told us that when we feel the breath in our body, it helps us feel, and open up. It also helps with touch. I liked feeling the touch of my breath in my body. Massaging my inner temple, and feeling how strong the breath is, compared to the mind. Knowing that past, present, and future thoughts are happening right here.

I am also finishing off my three day juice cleanse at Clover Juice which I was inspired to do, and I must say I feel a lot more energy. I feel lighter, and I noticed something during these three days of my juice cleanse, I have to juice more. I always resisted juicing because I wasn't ready. If you are being called to juice or try it, do it. The first couple of days I had my moments of temptation, and also on the first day had headaches caused by caffeine, but it passed after day one. I am amazed by what simple things do to your body.

In yoga, it is the breath and the pose (body) with the mind wanting to get in the way. When I am juicing it is the same thing, the breath and body, with the mind trying to intervene. So the practice for juicing is the same for yoga, be patient with yourself, be kind, be gentle within yourself, and most of all give yourself a break. Everyone works differently, and most take time to get it, with some moving slow and others fast, but you will get there, which is being present here.

I recommend Clover and the staff has been awesome and very helpful. I have done many fasts, but if you can, have someone guide you, it helps, trust me.

Day 51 of 90

"A" for Alice

Day 51 of 90 straight days of hot yoga at Moksha Yoga LA and I found myself with lots of energy after three days of drinking juice and water and feeling wonderful from the inside out. It has been hot out here in LA and so I rested a little longer outside in the lobby before entering the studio for practice. I walked in, lay on my mat and closed my eyes, continuing my intention from last night to start to incorporate a closed eye practice. So I spent about 50 percent of the practice with closed eyes. I am doing this to sense my breath and body more.

Teacher Alice entered class to guide our practice and her name would be easier understood as "A" my name is Alice, which of course is in reference to a musical, but in this case the "A" can be a reference to anatomy. She was amazing with the information she gave us including how to use the body and how the anatomy worked in each pose. It really helped me, in particular when I closed my eyes. I feel yoga should be done with eyes closed, so we release our identification with comparing, competing, and showing. The closed eyes have offered me a true sense of balance, and deeper trust. Life is here to support us. We are supported but we need to understand, practice, and engage the support within. Yes, my practice was wobbly with eyes closed, but the challenge was real, very real. I could sense so much within, that when my eyes are open in a pose and I am falling, I over-compensate to catch myself. With eyes closed, well you might want to yell, "Timber!" or "Man done down." With my eyes closed I am in complete trust of this moment, with no sense of where I am going, just here, just now.

I finished my juice fast at Clover Juice and feel great today, alive, and cleansed. It was short, but for a parent, with a daughter at home, it is perfect. If you are a parent and you are looking to do a short, fun, and healthy cleanse, I recommend this three-day cleanse. And then, from there, you can decide whether you want to continue. I very much enjoyed the different ingredients and how simple they were. There is nothing like sponsoring local farms and that makes me feel good, and it saves gas. The Black Chia is wonderful for cleansing you out and the Rev'd Up really gets your organs going. I love the green drinks for breakfast and dinner. Two thumbs up to Clover, and two thumbs up for me for listening!

Day 52 of 90

The "D" Word and Miracles

Day 52 of 90 straight days of hot yoga at Moksha Yoga LA and I relaxed in the lobby before entering class. I love sharing. Today I had a wonderful opportunity to talk with another man about his divorce and he shared how yoga saved him. The mind is funny, because when I heard divorce, my mind registered "Divine."

Divorce hit me hard and going through it at times felt like a very lonely experience. Looking back I probably went through periods of depression and anxiety. It felt like the wind got knocked right out me. I understand the word "divorce" can really scare people or the labels people put on it. So to hear "Divine" in place of divorce it allowed me to open up to a new inspired gift today. It would be wonderful if when going through a divorce, job loss, financial loss, health problem, and so on, if instead of labeling it with any of those words, we called it Divine.

It may look like this: "Hey David I thought you were married?"

And I would reply, "I was, but the Divine showed up and decided it was best to move in another direction for both of us."

The other person says, "Congratulations on the Divine showing up."

So today I looked at this experience on my mat as the Divine showing up and practicing. For when we say, "Namaste," are we are actually acknowledging the Divine in each of us. Teacher Grant was wonderful with the practice today, allowing us to use a block between our thighs to feel the inward pull of the thighs in our poses, and the strength of the inner muscles. He explained each pose and even demonstrating for us the right way to do them. When we pull into the body, go into our breath, we are acknowledging our real strength. Yoga is not about how bendy you are, or flexible, but if you can, allow the breath to express the pose. When it is all working you can't help but acknowledge the divine right where you are. The miracle you actually are. You have this breath, which is breathing you and us without judgment of your life, experience, or anything. That is beautiful, don't you think?

After class I went to Clover Juice and had a wonderful shake entitled CHIA SPA, good for hydrating and it had Omega in it and other great things. I love Clover it offers so many different things and today I had to toss a coin.

Day 53 of 90

For Courage

Day 53 of 90 straight days of hot yoga at Moksha Yoga LA and I entered today's practice with the intention of giving myself a gift. I spoke today and so afterwards it felt great to do yoga and let go. There is no better gift I can think of than taking the Yin class at Moksha. A restorative practice and especially going everyday now, it helps to just chill. I never know what will flow from me on my blog each day. I do the practice and on my walk home, things come up, and by the time I start to write, none of the things I thought about on the walk home come out in the blog. Funny.

I love teacher Emily and feel blessed she decided to follow her heart and come to LA. At the end of class she shared this beautiful poem, called "For Courage" by John O' Donohue. I felt it was good to share it, because you may feel fear coming up about something, and we all need courage sometimes. It has taken me courage to share this journey with you, it is taking courage for me to go 90 days, and then open my life up to you. As I do that, I understand that I am opening up to everything that may come, such as criticism, judgment, or support. But I have decided to stay open in my heart no matter what is happening, and never close down again. I closed down for a couple years, and frankly it stinks. I crawled up in a shell of guilt and shame, and it hurt. Stay open no matter what. So thank you for reading this book and cheering me on at Moksha, or sending me a kind email of support. So now I am going to enjoy my Black Chia from Clover. Enjoy your day as I move into day 54…Namaste

For Courage taken from
Benedictus: A Book of Blessings
By John O' Donohue

When the light around you lessens
And your thoughts darken until
Your body feels fear turn
Cold as a stone inside
When you find yourself bereft
Of any belief in yourself
And all you unknowingly
Leaned on has fallen
When one voice commands
Your whole heart,
And it is raven dark,
Steady yourself and see
That it is your own thinking
That darkens your world
Search and you will find
A diamond-thought of light,
Know that you are not alone
And that this darkness has purpose
Gradually it will school your eyes
To find the one gift your life requires
Hidden within this night-corner.
Invoke the learning
Of every suffering
You have suffered.
Close your eyes
Gather all the kindling
About your heart
To create one spark.
That is all you need
To nourish the flame

That will cleanse the dark
Of its weight of festered fear.
A new confidence will come alive
To urge you towards higher ground
Where your imagination
Will learn to engage difficulty
As its most rewarding threshold!

Poke at It

Happy Love Day! Day 54 of 90 straight days of hot yoga at Moksha Yoga LA and our teacher Matt was really cool, strong with the poses, and funny. I learned quite a bit about my practice and myself. On the way to practice I was aware of my inner dialogue, and then an image of Mountain pose came into my mind. As I became more aware of my body, I noticed that the voice in my head was nagging at me and I was being sucked into the nonsense; again an image of Mountain pose came forward, and the voice got louder, and my shoulders were forward, and lowering, and my whole front body was folding inward, as though I was being defeated. Again a picture of Mountain pose came in, I decided to follow the image. As I walked I brought my shoulders back and down, so my shoulder blades were resting behind the heart, this gently brought my heart up and out, with my heart expressing, my chin dropped slightly, allowing my neck to lengthen up, and guess what? No more inner dialogue. Done. I feel as if I pulled myself out of the lower abyss and into the higher planes.

So when class started, Matt our teacher told us of the image of Ganesh the elephant and that in some pictures Ganesh has a hook in his right hand. We are Ganesh, and we take the hook in life, poke at life and engage it, which is what I discovered I did on my walk over. So I decided that in my practice today, I would keep my heart open, like on my walk, and if my mind chatter started up, use that as a reminder to relax my shoulders and heart, and lengthen my neck. It was wonderful, this idea really helped me understand the need to pull in the stomach and then up in poses, it allowed my heart to drive. Matt our teacher reminded us after class to "poke life."

Day 55 of 90

I Am Alive

I walked into day 55 of 90 straight days of hot yoga at Moksha Yoga LA and my heart was open. Today my daughter started her journey at kindergarten. I sat there with her as she lined up with her classmates and started to tear up, followed by a flood of tears. My daughter gave me a huge hug and that was that. She waved goodbye and started her journey. I feel so blessed being there and being part of her life and showing up. So I lay down on my mat, closed my eyes and I think fell asleep. I'm not sure, but when I heard our teacher's voice welcome the class, my eyes shot open. Grant led us through a sweaty class of hot yoga. I was sweating just lying down today, and never stopped sweating. And as I am writing this I am still sweating. It was hot inside and out. Today I learned some adjustments in my shoulders and then I learned a valuable lesson on my mat. Let me see if I can simplify this.

So you come into an empty room in a house and you fill it with furniture. Every now and then you decide that you need to change the furniture around, because you yearn for change, but the empty room that you had is still the same, but filled with furniture. So now you spend time adjusting the furniture, but the space of the room remains the same. The only thing that is different is the furniture. But the space is the same. Do you see? We have all this space in us that we fill with our identity, thoughts, career, health, ideas, concepts and so forth, but the space is still there. The awareness is the space. We keep our identities and simply change the thoughts about it. So we don't really change. But we crave freedom, real freedom, and freedom is found in recognizing the space (awareness), and by recognizing the space we realize we are not the identity that we are clinging to.

I have been marching along on this journey of 90 days, and somewhere along the line I tried to move the furniture to keep up my identity; but that puts me in a loop, and that loop starts when I wake up in the morning and think – think that I know what will happen, or what is best for me, or plan my day. That produces the same outcome. There is no life to that. It is like being around a know it all, who knows nothing. It is true of the melodramatic mind. In the practice on the mat and off, I am called not to be sucked into the melodrama and to simply be aware of it. That is difficult sometimes, but it is the practice. So today I chose to feel everything inside me as I moved along today, and I realized that we have simply spent most of our lives moving the furniture around to protect us from feeling the heart. But the more I feel, the stronger I am now, and the more I am alive. So today on and off my mat was about experiencing life fully right now. When I do that, it takes away being right, or feeling wrong. And places me directly in the experience itself.

On to day 56...

Day 56 of 90

"Listen to Your Body"

Day 56 of 90 straight days of hot yoga at Moksha Yoga LA and yes it is quite warm here in LA-LA-Land. Today's practice was with teacher Joe and it was a class of flow – hey that came out like poetry. Over the past couple of days I have been doing a self-practice off my mat of witnessing the thoughts as they are, then noticing my body. If the thoughts are negative my body will fold forward, and collapse in. And when this happens, in order to break the cycle inward, I do Mountain pose. First I gently pull my shoulders back and down, which allows my heart to lift and chin to drop, I soften my heart and shoulders with my breath, and I am back in the clear.

So after doing this self-practice for a couple of days, I recognized that something was noticing the thoughts. Otherwise how would I know I have thoughts, unless they were being witnessed? So in recognizing this, "I" was witnessing the thoughts and so these thoughts can't be mine, unless I let them pull me in and then I become them. So simply by witnessing the thoughts, it gives more space inside and out.

Teacher Joe invited us to listen to our bodies. Today that became a little easier, because I could listen to the body, and then witness the thoughts wanting to make judgments on the sensations. This allowed the practice to meet the pose right where the body was, without getting caught up in what the mind was "thinking" about. Day 56 offered me the opportunity to sit in the pose and work where I am.

Foundation

Day 57 of 90 straight days of hot yoga at Moksha Yoga LA and getting closer to two months in. Wahoo! The community of Moksha is a wonderful family and very supportive. Today I had the opportunity to meet some new people whom I practice with quite a bit. It was fun meeting them. During my 57 days on the mat, I am seeing the importance of foundation. It has taken me quite a few falls, wobbles, and mistakes, finally to find proper foundation and I am still diving deeper into it. But at least I have a foundation to go to. I like the word foundation because it means, "Where something is supported." Each of us is looking for foundation in our life, through relationships with inner self, then with others, then with community, and then with the world community.

So today, in Carolina's class, I discovered through her flow class the support of each pose. Each pose offers support, alignment, strength, and most important our hearts. Each pose is an expression of the heart through the breath and then comes the expression through the body. So our support comes from within then moves out. The practice is feeling the support of the core, the spine, and legs grounded, with heart expressing up and chin down, feeling the inner energy of our inner temples. I noticed today on my mat that the breath is always moving me past my comfort zone, whereas the monkey mind just wants to be comfortable and okay all the time. The breath heart does not. It wants to explore past the past, and live here in the gift of the present.

So in my practice, when I focus on the movement of the breath, the foundation of the pose, all is flowing, then I am moved past my comfort zone, which is wonderful, because off my mat I can then live presently, allowing the flow of life to happen, without my mind dictating what to do. In the foreign film, *The Grandmaster*, a master is described as someone that does three things, "Being, knowing, and doing." We practice that on the mat. Being present. As we become more comfortable in not using the mind, then we can fall into the heart and listen to the breath of intuition. From there we will live from a place of knowing, and then our doing will become like an archer shooting a bow, focused, aligned, and laser like.

We will leave the comforts of doing all the time without purpose, and we will take that energy and focus it. Moksha is liberation. We are here to liberate ourselves as a community on our mats inwardly, and then express it outwardly, always living from the inside out!

Corpse Pose

Day 58 of 90 straight days of hot yoga at Moksha Yoga LA and this morning was filled with my daughter's school singing, and it was wonderful watching all the different expressions of kids. Today's practice was strong with moments of adjustment. I asked for help. I used to have trouble asking for help, as for some reason I had feelings of defeat, sometimes shame, or unworthiness that I couldn't do it. Now I realize that none of that is true. So if I need help, or have a question, guess what? I am asking.

Matt our teacher is a good, strong teacher. His demonstrations, and adjustments are really great. I connect really well to his guidance. I love being adjusted, especially now that I have been doing so many days back to back. I am starting to really understand what it feels like to have dominion over the mind and body, and allow the Divine to come through.

This morning I experienced a death meditation. In Buddhism a death meditation is to visualize yourself dying. First the ears go quiet, organs go, breath stops, and so on, and it continues with feeling the family clean your body, and then being put in a casket, and then feeling the dirt being thrown on you and finally being put in the ground. At no point in the meditation do you experience the death from outside yourself; you are in it.

What you realize, going through the process, is that at any point in your life you will breathe, and the breath won't come back. That is it, end of story. Your identity, sexuality, race, creed, salary, home, dogma, all the things and people you fought with, or were good with, gone. I do this to remind me of the preciousness of the moment. The fragility of the body and the power of the breath, without the breath, we are done. Death shows us that we are equal. We might differ in religion, God or no God, politics, sexuality, but death is what we go through, all of us, no escaping. It is real.

In Buddhism, death is the first thing that is looked at and confronted. If you run from death, you will be lazy, judgmental, arrogant, pride filled, controlling, greedy, you won't want to do spiritual practice all the time, you will want quick fixes, and you will expect people to play by your rules, until you sit with your death. Then it changes. Death brings you life. You see that by sitting with your death, you realize, you have no idea at all how long you will be here.

Then one day, death comes to you and says, "It's time." You explain, give me more time, and death says, "I gave you 24 hours in a day, seven days a week, and 52 weeks a year, and you did nothing, what will more time give you." If you get a chance, be with your death.

She-Ra

Day 59 of 90 straight days of hot yoga at Moksha Yoga LA and the journey continues. Today was filled with lots of reminders, and our teacher today Deena taught a wonderful class filled with great instruction, positivity, wisdom, and lots of encouragement. As I thought of our teacher, the name She-Ra kept coming to mind. Deena has a wonderful inner strength like a warrior, and mentioned to us, "Go beyond your habits to find stillness." I like that.

Today as I lay on my mat and set the intention to go past my comfort zone, I noticed in most of my poses I moved past my comfort zone and into a place of depth. It felt good to know that I could. Deena mentioned that the more present you are, the more you will discover you can. So in the practice the more engaged I am in each pose, the more I discover in my practice that my body, mind, and spirit are working as one, and all is quiet within. But when I am not fully focused in the pose, I do realize the likelihood of the mind wanting to come in to resist it, which reminds me to focus on the breath and breathe into the pose, and by doing that simple response, it brings me back fully into it.

Moksha means liberation and as I enter my mat every day, the intention is to liberate and free myself from the conditions that I have created. So every day is another day to release me from the habits Deena talked about today. And I choose to move past the habits, conditions, and fears, and as I do this, I move closer to the heart of being present in each pose and expressing more of a deeper self. That is encouraging and exciting as well.

Deena mentioned the opportunity we have to choose how we feel in each pose, and it is up to us how we feel, which is a wonderful lesson and invitation to explore how I show up off the mat as well.

Turned 60

Day 60 of 90 of straight days of hot yoga at Moksha Yoga LA and I showed up to celebrate milestone 60 by taking Yang/Yin with teacher Emily B. The first part of class is filled with flow and the later part is filled with restorative poses. Emily led us through a wonderful practice and reminded us of being with the pose. She offered us a couple moments to challenge ourselves, and even if we fell over, it didn't matter. I am learning there is always a moment when I can sense my growth. I must admit, growth happens all the time, but it is a process, and a patient one at that. Today I felt very strong in the flow and connected, and it was great to feel my inner strength and feel how much power is inside. I also listened to my body and listened to it without wanting to push through the pose.

There is a wonderful story of a bamboo plant, which grows five inches in five years and then, out of the blue, it grows nine feet. It shoots up nine feet tall. WOW! Pretty incredible; so sometimes it feels as if our growth isn't happening, or as if we aren't growing. But that is not true. Every day is a chance to show up on our mat and as we show up, we grow. Why? Because what I have learned is to just show up, be present, and be with the pose. Let the pose be the teacher and the breath the guide. Together they are learning to trust each other. Sooner or later they will have moments of unity. When that happens, it is hard to explain, and the only way I can, is that it is "AWEsome."

Day 61 of 90

Transitions

Day 61 of 90 straight days of hot yoga at Moksha Yoga LA and as I entered Moksha, I heard they are changing the name in the States to MODO. So soon you will read MODO YOGA not Moksha YOGA. Today as I entered practice, it was with a month to go until I reach 90. I am very grateful and appreciative of the support on FB, Twitter, Moksha, and messages on my email. I received this wonderful message from Sid on Saturday. "I'm loving your blog. It's like a daily vitamin for the soul." In this world of technology, sometimes we have no idea who is reading or seeing our work. So feedback is always wonderful to receive.

Today our teacher Joe focused on the breath as we moved through the Moksha practice. Our whole focus was breath, which may seem easy but in a 60-minute practice, with no music to distract you, well there can be places of challenge. What I noticed in the practice today may surprise you, maybe not – the breath continues to breathe and the only thing that seems to change beside the physical pose is the melodrama in the mind. So it is quite funny to notice when my breath stops because it is the melodrama in the mind getting in the way of the movement. But in actuality the only thing moving is the body from pose to pose. And the body is present, the breath is present, and the mind is looking to just be comfortable and okay all the time.

So the realization I had in the practice today was the recognition of the breath breathing for 60 minutes, the body moving, and the mind in melodrama mode. It feels good to feel the breath moving in the body. As you feel the breath in your body now, just become aware of it. I was also aware of the breath within myself and the room and how it was breathing each of us, giving the classroom life, and connecting us to our beingness. I feel we should change the word being to "Breathing." It would change a lot of drama within and without. Just picture it now, "I am a human breathing or a Spiritual Breathing." It changes the focus of how we see ourselves in others and others in us.

Day 62 of 90

Practice

Day 62 of 90 straight days of hot yoga at Moksha Yoga LA and we have a reminder of our daily practice. Whatever you choose to explore as your practice, whether it is ACIM, meditation, hiking, Pilates, Yoga, prayer, or repeating the Our Father, let it be a daily one. When we have a daily practice, we have a foundation, we have support, and we have something to go to when things are rolling along in our lives or falling over. If I have learned one important thing with practicing every day it is just that, practice, practice, practice. Practice is not so much about being perfect, as it is to help us surrender to the bigger self – the Divine.

I had the incredible opportunity last year of meeting Archbishop Desmond Tutu, and watching him speak to a crowd gathered at LACMA, for my good friend Robert Taylor's book signing. Someone raised their hand and asked the Archbishop about his thoughts on crime in Mexico, and what could he do about it. He smiled big, then laughed, and explained, "I laugh because you expect the Dalai Lama and me to do the work, and that is the problem, you don't want to do the work for yourself, so you throw money at it, and it is still there, so you put it on us. What can you do? We need you to do the work, we need you to pray, and meditate, take action." That is the importance for all of us to do the inner work. Not just do it and tell people about how spiritual we are or how we are not spiritual. This planet is given to us and we must take care of her. We do that through our practice first, and by taking care of us first, then our families, then the community, and then the planet. How you are affects the rest of us.

Today's practice with teacher Joe was a gift. The gift was to look at the importance of practice. Yoga to me is not about how flexible you are, or not. It is not about the fancy clothes, or how you look. Those are benefits of the practice. The gift of the practice is your connection to the whole self, the unity of mind, body, and spirit. That is an everyday experience. Yoga is inner work, inner play, which effects the alignment. Most poses turn inward, rotate inward, and it helps with the expression outward. I have noticed the practice become simple, subtle, and intuitive. When I show up on my mat, it is like a surgeon showing up for surgery. It is a skill, takes patience, breath, focus, and compassion for self.

Just like your practice. Practice is building a skill. Every skill takes patience, breath and compassion. Joe our teacher said today, "When you fall that is great, it means you are entering the unknown." Reminder: Practice, practice, and practice.

Day 63 of 90

The YES Machine

Day 63 of 90 straight days of hot yoga at Moksha Yoga LA and after experiencing a day that was non-stop busy, I showed up for the last class of the night, Yin, with teacher Katie. It was good to be back in one of Katie's classes, she has a warm presence and wonderful style of teaching. In class today I recognized that the breath is a constant yes machine, that it never stops saying yes to now. That the breath is constant, and the mind is the only thing that resists right now.

So on my walk home I sat with that thought, and it occurred to me that the breath knows that there is nothing that can't be done. Whether you are an athlete and under pressure, or a student taking an exam, or at work feeling stress, or sitting in traffic, what can you turn to? Your breath is the answer. The breath is so powerful that it can relax the mind in a crunch, it can relax the body in times of stress, and it can be used to simply meditate with.

In Yin practice tonight I was in awe of the beauty of the breath. It really is quite amazing. It is like the breath knows the answer is here, it also knows that the answer will come forward in patience, in relaxation, and when we are not focused on the problem. Because the breath is never focused on the problem, the breath is happening now. Sit with the breath now. Just be aware of the breath moving in your body, moving with ease and grace, and notice how when you are thinking it stops the breath. Thinking gets in the way of the one thing giving you life, your breath. What is wonderful about this is it teaches all of us that we are not "Human thinkers" or even "Spiritual Thinkers," but we are "breathing" which is "Being".

Today's practice was a wonderful reminder of the true power

of allowing the breath to guide us and rest here as it is. Because really what is there to defend, but out dated habits. When we control people, situations, and life, we are selfish. So practice allowing the breath and also contemplating the breath and see where it takes you

Day 64 of 90

You are Right Here

Day 64 of 90 straight days of hot yoga at Modo Yoga (the name has now changed) and what a perfect class for me to take. My day had already revealed some surprises to me, and so hearing Joe start class with, "You are where you are right now. You are always in the perfect place." With those words something came forward, a new mind set. I have been writing about the body and breath, both of which are here on the mat. There is only really one thing that is refusing to accept "now," and that is the mind. Joe reminded us that we are connected to the people next to us, that being mindful of stillness affects those around us and is quite powerful. I am discovering the nobility in stillness. Joe brought up that the mind needs to put attention on something and so he invited us to put it on the breath. What was wonderful was the realization of, "Okay I am right here, nowhere else," and then came this wonderfully strong practice, fully present and expressing. I could feel the person on my right, and behind me, and in front me, I could feel their energy, as we were there for each other.

At one point I went beyond my comfort zone, and fell over, and my first thought was not "Shame on you for falling," but the first thought was, "Awesome, David, you went past what you knew and tried something different." Everything felt stronger today, alive, engaged, and opened. Flow was fun and exciting. I could really sense the power of community, of life itself, of yoga, of expressing fully with no boundaries.

Courage

Day 65 of 90 straight days of hot yoga at Modo Yoga and I discovered that the breath is the drumbeat of the spirit, and the heart is the vision. In yoga practice as we move together as a class, we move like the inner workings of the body. Everyone is playing a part and each part matters to the whole.

Today, in practice, teacher Joe led us through a vigorous flow, followed by a restorative practice. Joe always has wonderfully insightful things to teach us on our mats. Today was no different. In the practice I discovered how hard I had been working with my feet, and relaxed them down; and, as I did that, I discovered the four parts of the foot and I realized I could surrender the feet to the ground. I noticed that everything in yoga is happening now. This may seem like a "duh" moment, but in practice when the focus is here, and we are not worried about what just happened, or about how it looks, or where we are headed, then the flow of the pose is natural.

A good example of this is the chin. The chin represents faith in some energy work. So by dropping the chin and allowing the rise of the back of the neck, we become relaxed here, and more trusting of the present, but in one of the poses I was pushing my chin out. Joe acknowledged that and reminded me to bring the chin in. As I did I noticed how important it is not to push through poses. So balance on the mat is subtle, and awareness is important in each pose. It is easy to push through things, but resting here, where you are is just as important.

Restorative poses reminds me of the journey, the journey of being with the experience as it is unfolding. As we move with the experience that life presents to us, sometimes we have lots of pain we are moving with; therefore, wanting to get to the end of it by pushing through it so we can show people how strong we are, is how most people live.

When people come to me for sessions, most of the time they are moving through death, crisis, big emotions, and life circumstances, and they meet with me to heal; but most people believe there is a quick fix, a switch, a big tool, to magically rid them of the feelings. There is not. What there is though is being with the experience as it is happening. As you do, you build the heart of warrior. Every time you move through things on your mat and off, you become stronger; you might not see it right away, but you will see it. But first you must have the willingness to be with it. That is difficult. Joe reminded our class, "Have the courage to change."

Emotions when fully experienced only last for 45 seconds to a minute, but when the mind story kicks in, and the emotions are not fully experienced they can last from a day to 50 years. That is why being on your mat matters – to build your courage to be with the experience, and to know inwardly that you can handle life as it is, and as it is presented to you.

Challenges, Adjustments, and Changes

Day 66 of 90 straight days of hot yoga at Modo Yoga and as I move closer to day 90, I was reminded of patience and focus. Today our class was taught by Emily M, and it was really great. My mom loves watching strong women on screen and in life, and I bring that up because of the strong women teachers here at Modo Yoga. All are really strong, disciplined, and filled with wisdom. Today was no different. As we entered the studio for practice, Emily M offered us an invitation to pick a place in the studio we have never been and place our mats down there. Simple? Maybe.

I realized in my practice how often I practice around the outer parts of the room, and never put myself in the center of the room. Well today I plopped down in the center room, and I felt uncomfortable, so I sat with it on my mat before class and felt it, and it went away. It is amazing, and is as Emily pointed out, "How we create habits and get stuck in them." The challenge I had in the practice today was my body just felt tight and stuck. So it felt great to have Emily give me some slight adjustments and challenge me to go further. When she did, I went further. By going further, the tightness and stuck feeling went away.

This is why I love this practice, or any practice, the more you show up, the more opportunity you will have to be fully focused on the mat and trust the practice in bringing you past your edge. I realized afterwards, that I was beginning to get comfortable in the poses, so by having Emily adjust me, I was able to expand my edge and work through some tough aspects of my own practice. This reminds me of love, as we weed away all the stuff that keeps us from fully loving.

Emily spoke about the challenge of slowing down in the

practice and how when we do that, the mind picks up. So she offered us the invitation to allow the thoughts to come and to go away. To the strong women out there and heart-centered men – keep shining!

Two Roads

Day 67 of 90 straight days of hot yoga at Modo Yoga and the morning started bright and early. I was a guest on the radio show called, *Love by Intuition Show* hosted by Deborah Beauvais. The radio show is in Boston and I was talking about my 90-day yoga journey, the importance of the heart, and much more. What a great way to start a morning and I felt very blessed by the experience. When the show ended, she asked what my day looked like, and I said, "Well I am off to day 67 of 90."

So I arrived at Modo Yoga and took Grant's class, and used the example from yesterday's class, to continue to find a new place in the room to practice. Today I planted myself in the front row, took my shirt off, and faced the mirror. As I looked at my reflection I saw my Mountain pose eyes, a soft heart, and a man who had inner strength. Something between yesterday's practice and today shifted. Perhaps it was Emily M guiding me past my comfort zone, and perhaps by doing that yesterday, something clicked inside, a shift within, an acknowledgement of who I am on the mat and off. I am not my thoughts, my identities, but I am that which is always present now – awareness.

During Grant's class we had many opportunities to look at ourselves in the mirror and to check our alignment, and over and over I noticed how strong, grounded, and heart opening I looked. If this reads like it shocked me, it did. For the first time today I could really see my inner transformation in my eyes. Grant challenged us today to go into the breath and allow the breath to take us deep into the pose. What I love about yoga is the more you practice, the more you really relish the moments of no movement, just breathing, just rest, and how enlightening it is to sense the power of Shavasana (Corpse Pose) at the end of practice.

Class starts, just like life, connecting into your breath, and you move through the poses, just like your life. One moment you feel like standing still in Mountain pose, the next you move into Warrior 1 then Warrior 2, some days you are twisted up in Tree pose, and some days you are falling over like a toppling tree. All the while in life on the mat and off, we are taught to meet the experience where we are now, then just like the yoga practice, life ends in Shavasana. The "you" that walked in has died and been made anew. Grant made reference to this death of us in our practice.

I love the poem "Two Roads" by Robert Frost:

"Two roads diverged in a yellow wood, and I—
I took the one less traveled
And that has made all the difference."

The road less traveled to me is the road within. It is difficult for many people to go inward. My hope is that this blog inspires you to go there, feel there, live in there, because you might not be able to change the war, or the violence out there, but you can choose to change it inside.

Tao of Dave

It is day 68 of 90 straight days of hot yoga at Modo Yoga, and in practice today I was inspired by a gentleman practicing on my left side. It was his first time practicing, and he was probably around 70 years old and he was taking the flow class. I came out and told him after class that he was, "Rad." That is right, rad! I loved it!

On one side of me I had a gentle old man, who was taking each pose as it was and as he could deal with it, breath by breath; on my right side I had a buffed gentleman who was very physical, and willful. I was in the center. Over these past 68 days, pretty much every teacher has mentioned that we are here in class as a community, that we pick each other up, that we can feel each other, and today was the class I could feel the energy of both people. It was quite powerful to feel the subtle energy of the man to my left, and then to my right to feel willful energy of strength and power. To be in the center of that, was to understand the middle ground within.

We are taught in Modo Yoga to breathe into things, it helps in relaxing the body, and it also signals to the body and mind that we can handle it. So I have noticed in my two days with Grant, the middle ground of my practice taking over, which is showing up in my life off the mat as well. Someone mentioned something to me the other day, and I would have taken off into some emotional melodrama at what they said, but I was aware of the comment, and their intention as well, so I acknowledged it, felt it, and took a breath right into it. That led me to a choose point, and I chose to let go and move on. I felt the breath disable the old program and create a new program. I love the new program. The new program responds, not reacts. The new program takes action, and no longer constantly is in a loop of doing. Action is focused and centered in breath awareness.

Grant offered us an opportunity to play in some poses, and it felt good to play in my core strength, allowing the full energy to be focused and scattered about.

21 days

Day 69 of 90 straight days of hot yoga at Modo Yoga and I found myself in a flow class with teacher Matt. I like Matt's no BS style of teaching as it cuts right to the core and to the point. Today in class we focused on the deepening of the pose and adding some twists, along with lots of flow. The practice was filled with flow and instruction. Matt has been speaking on the Ganesh holding a poker, a noose, and an ax. They are symbols for our practice. We poke at where we want to go, then we put a noose around it, and we use the ax to free ourselves from what we choose.

When I started this journey on the mat, I chose to experience holding on to the past, and it feels lately I took an ax to that idea, and now I am poking at my greatness, my heart, and liberation, all of which can only happen here.

In the practice today I found lots of strength breathing into my belly, and when I looked into the mirror it looked like a Buddha belly hanging over my yoga pants. I noticed the belly pulling up naturally in poses, and also noticed my Down Dog pose finally found the ground. My heels had finally reached the ground and so for the first time in my practice my foundation was cemented in. I can tell you that this feeling of being grounded to the earth and then expressing in the pose makes a world of difference. Even my Three-legged pose was strong.

As I continue to unravel my heart and trust in it more, my practice is becoming stronger, grounded, and patient. The hard edges have fallen away, the part that lived in constant worry has burned up, and the song, "Don't worry be happy," actually makes perfect sense, "Don't worry," why create the worse outcomes? Why imagine the worst? Why not just choose to be happy? Who cares if it all goes away? You can still be happy. You can be happy with nothing or a lot.

I told someone today who was in panic mode, "Remember this, one day you will breathe, and the breath will not come back. So will this really matter then?" They stopped, and smiled, and acknowledged me with, "Point taken." Some people are too busy dying, rather than living now. But when you are present, the action is simple. Worry makes things too complicated. Fear is complicated. The truth is simple. Things happen. The breath comes in and goes out, the rest is just a narrative and in the narrative we put a noose on ourselves, and forget we put it there. So acknowledge it and choose to free yourself.

Holy Moly 70

Day 70 of 90 straight days of hot yoga at Modo Yoga and I woke up at 4:30 am for a 6 am class today. As I awoke from my slumber, I thanked the Divine for another day of life, another day to practice, another day to love fully, and another day to be of service. How blessed are each of us. When we drop the need to worry, we can see the blessings of right now.

Today marks day 70, "Holy Moly." When I started this I was just going for 30 straight days, now I am on day 70, and what a journey. All of us are amazing. There is a wonderful song by Master Sha that starts with, "I love my heart and soul, and I love all humanity." I am reminded of that now. Say that today, reflect on that, "I love my heart and soul."

Today I celebrated day 70 with a flow class with teacher Carolina. She is always a great example of inner strength and instruction. Her style is clear, strong, and compassionate. I learn quite a bit about myself in her class, especially at 6 am.

Today I learned that I am truly grateful for the practice today, grateful for the work I have for today, grateful to coach my first practice with 16 under-eight girls in soccer, grateful for my light filled daughter, my parents, my family, all my teachers, friends, for Modo Yoga, and for all the support people have given me in emails, comments, and on the street on this yoga journey. And so grateful that the Divine has given me life today to breath it all in to my heart. Grateful that no matter what happens in our life or how it looks, that we can do it, move through it, and although it may take time, sooner rather than later, we will see the light of why it unfolded as it did. But right now be with it, be with life, as it is moving through you.

A woman saw me in Trader Joe's yesterday and smiled and

said, "Congratulations on your yoga journey, you are so inspiring." The Divine always finds the right time to speak to us through others and remind us of how special each of us really is. Yes, we all matter, each of us. Now there will be people who will say you don't matter, silently bless them and move on. There are people on this planet that can't wait to see you, love you, and be around you, because they love you as you are. Go to them. Give up making others wrong to be right, give up changing anyone, give up pettiness, putting guilt on others, shaming or humiliating others, or fixing anyone (when they are ready they will ask for help), until then, just be of service. Service comes from worthiness, knowing that you are loved and love itself expressing. Service – being still and happy are noble acts, the highest acts one can live. Even when things are falling apart, choose stillness, choose service, and choose to be happy.

It Begins With You

Day 71 of 90 straight days of hot yoga at Modo Yoga and today's class taught by Emily B was wonderful. She shared with us about the day of peace on September 21st, and asked us to contemplate, "What does peace mean to you?" I have been asked this question a couple times, in classes, and at services, and my answer today really surprised me, "Acceptance." So I used that as my intention for class today.

Emily also invited us to make peace with ourselves. Every day that I have been practicing on the mat, I step closer to that treaty within; I step closer to peace. Because every day on the mat I am called to accept myself right where I am. A couple of days ago I might have had the practice of a lifetime, then the next day I show up and feel sluggish, what I have noticed with acceptance is that it helps me with everything.

Let's say I am fighting with myself inside, the moment I become aware it, I simply label it, "fighting," and it goes away. In class I had a moment of reflecting, so I was aware of it, and labeled it, "reflecting" it fell away. In some circles people will say, "let go" or "surrender" and those words I have a tough time with. But when I accept everything as it is, it helps in releasing my hold on them. In another moment in class I had a strong sensation in my hip, I felt it, and said to myself softly, "sensation." The sensation fell away, and it allowed more breath to seep into the space where the sensation appeared to be congesting the hip. As the breath entered the area of the hip I was able to expand more and deeply with grace.

Peace is an invitation to accept. Emily read a beautiful quote on peace, which was about having peace in our heart even with the noise happening. Peace, love, and harmony can only begin with each of us. Otherwise they are just words we throw around, but when those words become real to you inside, and you begin to feel the power in them, and the responsibility that comes with it, then life changes. We begin to watch how we use our words, how we treat others, how we respond to life, and how we treat ourselves; there is great importance to resolve the war inside now on this planet, and it simply begins with a choice to make peace inside. Break bread with our enemies and forgive them. Mother Earth is dependent on us now, more than ever.

Finding Peace When it is Hard

Day 72 of 90 straight days of hot yoga at Modo Yoga and today entering class I was feeling weighed down – not by anything really, just the day itself. So I lay on my mat and focused on the breath, allowing the day to fall away. And as practice began, what I felt had fallen away, had not. My practice felt like work, the body felt heavy, and the legs were wobbly. So through my practice of acceptance, I accepted where I was at, which helped loosen some things up. But overall, today the practice was heavy.

Teacher Emily B was wonderful, sharing a story of snowboarding, and strapping us in for the ride. Now what I noticed is when the practice feels almost like a grind, the easy path is to beat yourself up, but yoga is about acceptance, and acceptance is gentleness and compassion, which starts with us.

So when I felt myself wanting to push through, I labeled it, "pushing" and the pushing went away. In every single spiritual practice, whether we know it or not, the reason why we beat ourselves up is because we begin to see that it is happening inside us, and rather than be with the experience, we negate it, and when you negate something, it is easier to harm, punish, or hurt. It is why people judge and criticize others; it negates the person, and gives them permission in their mind to harm with judgments, hurts, or punishment. All control is selfish and lacks love.

It happens in the politics of war. We negate a country, which gives us permission to judge it, hurt it, and bomb it. By negating we dehumanize something. And we realize that there is no one to blame anymore, which can be frustrating, and we feel like we "should" be past this, or "this again!" But none of it is true. We just don't want to accept what is, so it is subtle. The mind takes us out of the experience, and then breath puts us back in and says, "Yes, David, this where we are; now receive the breath and give it away." So I just started a mantra, "I receive the breath" on the inhale and on the exhale, "I give it away." Simple.

I was happy I was able to be with it, even though I discovered the mind wanting to be perfect, and not wanting to accept. I refused to negate and dehumanize myself. Every spiritual practice humbles us. Today was humbling. Day 72 reminds us to "Receive the breath and give it away." Again thank you to Emily B for her constant guidance and reminders in class...

Peace Be With You

Day 73 of 90 straight days of hot yoga at Modo Yoga and I entered the studio awaiting a special class today in honor and the celebration of peace. Today is International Day of Peace. The class was a Yin class on Peace, facilitated by our teacher Emily B, and in the class she read poems, quotes, and we chanted OM, and listened to music, all with the intention of bringing peace inside.

Sometimes on my mat, in practice, an idea will come that will really catch my heart, like a dream catcher, catches dreams, and my heart is an inspiration catcher. What came to my heart was the idea of R.I.P. – Rest in Peace. The majority of people wait until they actually die to experience peace, why wait to experience peace when you die, why not experience it now, by learning meditation, yoga, Tai Chi, prayer, breathing, or anything that will facilitate in you, or as Emily put it, "Your own peace treaty."

There is a wonderful story Wayne Dyer used to tell of a man on his deathbed, and he turned to his wife and said, "What if I never lived my life fully?" Then he died. Another wonderful story is the ancient Egyptians believed that upon death they would be asked two questions and their answers would determine whether they could continue their journey in the afterlife. The first question was, "Did you bring joy?" The second was, "Did you find joy?"

I have sat with people dying, their eyes go clear, the heart expands, and weight is lifted off them. This same experience happens with waking up from your inner slumber. Today's class was a beautiful reminder of a famous Buddha story. When the Buddha started to wander around India shortly after his enlightenment, he encountered several men who recognized him to be a very extraordinary being. They asked him, "Are you a god?"

"No," he replied.

"Are you a reincarnation of god?"

"No," he replied.

"Are you a wizard, then?"

"No."

"Well, are you a man?"

"No."

"So what are you?" They asked, being very perplexed.

Buddha simply replied, "I am awake."

Buddha means "the awakened one." How to awaken is all he taught.

After taking several classes with most of the teachers, I love in Emily B's classes that under her breath, when she feels the class is doing well, in an almost whisper she says, "Good." I feel my guardian angels are like that. When I am present with things, even when the noise is a lot, if I acknowledge to myself this simple statement, "Yes, here is noise, and I am okay," I feel my guardian angels smile, and say, "Good."

Today examine in your life how you are with peace inside, and where you go when the noise seems relentless. Because I can promise you, peace is present with you. Practice peace. Love on you! Peace is with you.

The Question?

Day 74 of 90 straight days of hot yoga at Modo Yoga and I walked in and took a class right away. It was a straight Modo class that lasted 75 minutes. Our teacher was Grant and the class really focused on the breath and breathing into the pose. What a great reminder on a Sunday and the first day of fall. Fall is a wonderful reminder to go within and contemplate. We have created a world story where defense is the intention.

We defend our cars, homes, businesses, countries, lives, and we go to the doctor's and they look for what is wrong. Most people are always trying to fix, control, and manipulate others, all so we can feel safe and comfortable. Our language when we meet new people is geared toward asking, "What is wrong? Are you okay?" Or checking in, "How are you doing?" Most people never ask for prayer when things are going good, only when things seem to be going wrong.

Taking practice today on the mat, I looked at what is right in the practice. I looked at being with right now – experiencing the ever changing now. Every breath is different, every moment offers a new experience, and as we awaken from the slumber, we notice the mind is always in defense of itself. Defending the need to be right, the need to know, the need to attack, the need to need, and if we are not conscious of this, we will never uncover the mirage which keeps us from the presence. The mirage is subtle and loud. The mirage creates fear.

So in our yoga practice, the mirage can complain about the feelings inside the body, scream because the sensations are too much, the mirage can make us believe that these feelings are because of the outside, the mirage can force us to push through things because we are uncomfortable with how things are now, and the mirage can suggest thoughts that are completely untrue and want us to believe them as true. All to keep us from experiencing now. Pretty clever, and if we don't watch it, we become the cleverness, the manipulators, the controllers, the greedy, the haters, and so on. So waking up is most important. Not waking up our partners, families, the world, and making them wrong, but waking up us and becoming an example for our families, friends, strangers, and the world. That matters, because waking up matters. We are here to know ourselves. Not know other people's business and get involved.

So ask, "How am I being right now?" Be honest with yourself. Then be there.

BOA

Day 75 of 90 straight days of hot yoga at Modo Yoga and I found myself in Grant's class. Grant suggested as practice that we start to follow the breath and allow the movement. No matter how you cut it, the simpler things appear, the harder we make them. Another thing Grant told us was simply to notice the sensations, the body, in the practice. Over the past 75 days the same mantra has come forward, breathe, allow, and observe. Or simply we can call it BOA, breath, observe, allow.

I am always amazed by the power of breath, and that you can't hold it that long until the breath wants in or out. The breath is like water, it flows. It flows into the sensations and washes over them, it flows into resistance and relaxes it, and it flows into the practice, into life, into everything. Observe it now. Observe the breath, your own breath. Right now. Don't try to breathe, or will the breath, just observe it. To me observing is like being in a state of AWE. Your breath is AWE-some.

Today's practice on the mat was just that a practice. Every day on the mat is a practice, and in any spiritual practice we practice to simplify. Life is an experience. That is why in Zen they remind us, "Take out the laundry and do wash before enlightenment, after enlightenment take out the laundry and do wash." We are already love, peace, compassion, and inner strength and these qualities haven't left us, but the clouds of thoughts try to convince us that we are not the observer, but the thoughts themselves. So every day we set out to rest here, and as we rest, we recognize that there is noise in our head and it is just that, noise in our head. And there noise outside of us, it is just that, noise. So every day in our practice we forgive others and ourselves for trespassing, just like the Our Father suggests.

What is trespassing? For myself on my mat when I beat myself up that is trespassing against who I am. If I judge another, condemn, put down, punish, use my words to hurt rather than uplift another soul then I am trespassing against myself, and the other. So I must forgive. And know that it is okay, that I believed the noise was true, and it wasn't.

So today practice BOA – Breath-Observe-Allow.

Mother Mary

Day 76 of 90 straight days of hot yoga at Modo Yoga with teacher Carolina. My first book I ever wrote was never published it was entitled *Mary and Me*, and it was my dialogue with Mother Mary. I remember a section in the book where Mary said, "David, let the practice be to contemplate your breath." That terrified me because I had an active thinking mind and wondered how could focusing on your breath solely help? What about prayer and meditation? And she said, "David, the breath is the movement of God, it is answered prayer, it is meditation; words – no matter how beautiful they are can't capture God."

I bring that up because teacher Carolina asked us to deepen our breath and allow the breath to guide us. The moment you lose the moment you have lost the movement of the breath. Again this sounds simple but we move in a society of distraction. We are distracted from our peace of mind. Distracted by what we see, hear, and yet in the breath we become. We are always becoming. The breath, as Mother Mary told me, is everything. Practice that. Words are limiting, and experience is limitless.

We always want to describe our life with words, but words limit it. Texting can't express you, email can't, this blog can only offer a glimpse, TV can't do it, but in your breath, you can experience something called wonderment and awe.

Life is beautiful. Practice observing the breath and feel it in you. Stop wanting everyone to make you comfortable, to feel comfortable, life wants to expand, express, grow, and life is always on the cusp of death. Life is not comfortable. A tree is always growing, losing leaves, and gaining new ones. If your spiritual practice is about comfort than you will never grow.

Spirit (Breath) wants to soar. So follow the breath. See where it takes you.

Yoga is unification of breath, body, and mind as one movement.

The Offering

Day 77 of 90 straight days of hot yoga at Modo Yoga and I am reminded today at 6 am practice that every day we are offered another day to live on this planet. At night when we close our eyes, that could be it. When you wake up, it is easy to jump into habits that protect us from experiencing life in a new way. So as I walked to practice I embraced the breath, and thanked the Divine for allowing me this day. When I entered practice taught by Grant, and lay on my mat, I realized yoga is about the journey of meeting the Divine on the mat. This is our one-on-one time. No BS. No Escape. No proving. No needs. No wants. Just here and dealing with what comes up. And frankly it may not be comfortable. Life is not meant to be comfortable, but that does not mean you have to struggle with it, or even struggle.

This morning, for about a quarter of the practice, I was nagged by sweat and heat, and wanted to scratch and wipe the sweat away, and it was intense. But I was with it, and I don't know when, but those sensations that were nagging me fell away. Then I experienced intense memories coming up. Then that fell away. So yes, I am on day 77 straight of hot yoga, but it is just like day one, every day on the mat – like each day of life offers us a chance to ride the wave of life, go with the flow of it.

Grant offered us a moment of just sitting in meditation and observing the parts of the body. It felt great. Today you are offered another day to live. Live it presently here. See what happens.

Day 78 of 90

Modo Yoga

Day 78 of 90 straight days of hot yoga at Modo Yoga and again I found myself waking up early for the 6 am practice, this time with teacher Carolina. Carolina offered us the idea of just being here. We opened practice with sitting meditation and then went into Modo practice. It is great to shake it up. I loved having time to sit and sit in stillness before practice. From there we set our intention. For some reason the intention that came forward for me was "giving."

Without questioning the word "giving" as my intention, I dove in. In today's practice I found some subtle things happening. The "giving" turned out to be about allowing the breath to give to me and so I allowed the breath to go into my back area, fill up my kidneys, my spine, and I noticed I had fuller breaths. So the "giving" intention allowed for more life energy to flow into my body, which is wonderful, because normally when I wake up so early, I allow coffee to flow into my body, which is still fun.

I also noticed in our back bends today my breath was helping me in the pose by pulling me up and expanding along with my abs. So the breath and core were really starting to work as one, giving me strength, no longer using the mind in anyway. Imagine if you focus on the breath, and on each inhale it was as though it was giving you a gift, how abundant you would feel. Here we are looking for abundance out there in the world, and it is coming into our lungs all day long.

Honestly I can't believe I am on day 78 of 90 straight days. At soccer practice last night, one of my soccer moms said she was reading my blog and how it is helping her appreciate life and her breath. Very cool.

Today I felt inspired by the simplicity of breath and what a wonderful gift it is for all of us. The breath has no judgment and it breathes all of us equally. Like the sun shines on us all! Life is what is.

Day 79 of 90

The Tide

Day 79 of 90 straight days of hot yoga at Modo Yoga and as I entered the studio I met two groovy Vancouver Mokshies, Julia and Eric. Welcome to LA! Today I entered the studio with just a little over ten days to go, and give a thank you to all the people from all over the place for their tremendous support and that are sensing I am getting close. I am well supported and loved on this journey and I accept and receive it humbly. I took teacher Joe's class and it was a wonderful reminder of several things. First, we celebrate and support each other in class as a community of breathers, and, as always, Joe reminded us of our breath. Joe has great wisdom and love for life and yoga.

In class, as I was practicing, I noticed my breath, and it reminded me of the tide. Coming in and going out gently. I also noticed that if I push in any way, the breath shows me that I am pushing, by pounding the breath, just like the ocean in a storm pounding the beach. It helps me to notice the breath in this way, like I would the ocean. I am also aware that the only thing that stops the breath is thought, and when I am thinking in a pose, I am not breathing, I am holding on to the breath, holding on to the thoughts, because I am not trusting the experience as it is.

But when the breath moves like the tide, I begin to notice the subtleness and grace of yoga. In each pose, when I fully breathe, I can sense the hips gently moving in place, the foundation strong in them, and the actual movement of yoga happening. This is important, because foundation is important. The foundation is the breath. As yogis we are practicing to live fully here. I like to look at it in this way: we are practicing to "B.E." which means BREATH EXPERIENCE. Yoga is simply breath experience. Without thought, we have full union of breath, body, then mind, and it is all working together with the breath.

Each pose is just that, a pose with breath. The mind sees it differently. The mind sees the pose at first as a threat to its identity and panics. The breath comes to relieve the panic, and relax into it. So we do this dance of panic and relax for a while, until one day, we begin to trust the breath experience. Then each pose is simply a breath experience with twists, bends, flow, and stretching. It is no longer about being shallow and impressing people with our flexibility. Impressing means, I AM PRESSING, showing off. Yoga is about the breath experience.

Day 80 of 90

Day 80

Day 80 of 90 straight days of hot yoga at Modo Yoga and I felt very relaxed and deep in breath. The breath is the leader of the practice. Great leaders lead quietly and listen alertly, which is what we can say about our breath, it leads quietly.

Today teacher Grant led us through a practice that was about the breath and stillness. Between some of the poses we acknowledged the stillness and then moved on. This really allowed us to acknowledge the leader, which is the breath on the mat. The pose is the pose. The mind makes an interpretation of what it thinks is going on and it is almost always wrong. The breath is always safe and comfortable. It need not defend itself from attack, like the mind. The mind resists and the breath accepts. The difference is felt, not thought about.

Today marks day 80 of 90 straights days, and as I move closer to 90, the breath is becoming more and more prominent in my practice. In fact because the breath is leading now, I am more aware how important our words are off and on the mat. Will my speaking improve the moment or harm it? I am speaking to the speaking inside the body and outside. So the stillness we are moving in on our mat is whole and perfect. Our practice is perfect right now, no matter what it looks like. The breath leads. All is well, all is very well right here.

The mind cannot believe what I am telling you now as it has no capability to know what I am saying. But the breath knows all is well. The breath is safe as it flows with the flow of life, just like the ocean, each wave moves with it, without resistance. So today we allow the breath to lead.

81 is Fun

Day 81 of 90 straight days of hot yoga at Modo Yoga and I entered practice today with a little humility. During this process of practice I have been taking it one day at time. If I think of the number of days, it throws me off. So it has been quite humbling to practice every day, and the challenge off my mat has been balancing my life with a practice every day, but I have done it. I have done it because I have learned having a practice of any kind matters. When things go another way or life changes direction, I have something to go to, which will remind me of who I am in the middle of all of this. During the 81 days I have learned the importance of breathing; not so much through anything, but with it, and to accept everything as it is including the sensations, feelings, thoughts, and everything as it is. By practicing this way on my mat and off it has allowed many things to flow on by.

Today my practice was with teacher Carolina, it was a wonderful flow class filled with lots of reminders. At one point we were lying down and she reminded us to just let it all go. Funny how difficult it is, because when this life is over, we will have to let it go. And we won't have a choice in the matter. I find it empowering to have the choice to let it go now. I choose to let it go and let it flow. Why hold on? Why do we hold on to anything or anybody? And does the answer matter. The breath holds on to nothing.

Look at all the stuff that you think matters in your life, and ask yourself why? Why does the past matter? Why does the future matter? Why does what others say matter? Why do our thoughts matter so much? What is thinking? What is a thought? Who is noticing the thoughts? We spend so much time rushing around, avoiding the present moment that we miss it. We miss the only thing that really matters to us. The only place where change is natural and normal, we act as if change is an intrusive thing. It is not. Change is normal.

I discovered in practice today the opportunity to follow what Bruce Lee said, "When you punch, you punch not with your right hand; the punch comes from the whole being." So now when I practice, I practice to be full in every pose, give my fullness to it. Breathe into it, expand, and celebrate my being now. Yoga is life.

What Would Happen?

Day 82 of 90 straight days of hot yoga at Modo Yoga and this is a practice. Each of us is practicing life. Every day we are given the opportunity to express our hearts desire. Every day we are given another day of life. Yoga gives us that opportunity to accept everything as it is, and then make adjustments. Sometimes the adjustments are subtle, and sometimes they are big. But yoga teaches us on our mat to listen to the breath, follow it, trust it, and go into it. And yoga does it in safe environment.

Matt facilitated today's practice and I like his no BS approach to yoga. Just get in there and experience it. Simple. Yoga is about experiencing life as it is. This is not easy. We resist everything when we live in the monkey mind. Today I find myself in the living breath. Your breath is alive, and it gives you life, what more do you need?

Matt taught us through practice today many twists; and what I gathered from that, on my mat, is life offers us many twists and turns, so can you breathe with them. Not through them, or push them away, or run, or hide, or make stories, excuses, or even worry, but can you breathe with them as they are and trust that the answer will come. Not on your time frame but with the flow of life itself. Nature meets every need effortlessly, and we are taught to struggle with everything. Why? Why is it so difficult to just accept things as they are? Why do we judge them, criticize them? What are we scared about? What will happen if you actually trust in the flow of life? Trusting in the flow is really just accepting life right where you are.

Can you imagine just accepting everything in your life as it is, people, circumstances, situations, etc…everything as it is? Sit with that. What would happen? There would be nothing left to fix or change in anyone. Life is not so much about fixing, changing, because life does that naturally. Nature balances everything out. So does life. So live life with a good heart, forgive, and accept. Keep it simple.

Conan the Barbarian

Day 83 of 90 straight days of hot yoga at Modo Yoga LA and I showed up early expecting to wait around to take teacher Joe's class, but since I got there early, I went into teacher Grant's class whom I call "Conan the Barbarian," frankly because he looks like "Conan the Barbarian." Grant's style is wonderful to practice to. He has shifted to lots of reminders of the breath, helping us relax in the stillness, and ending practice with meditation. I am glad that I showed up early. Yesterday I did a morning practice and a night practice, which were both flow classes. Today was a Modo class. Within in two minutes I was sweating. This class had no music, except for the music of our breath. In yoga our muse is the divine breath, breathing each of us.

One cool thing about a hot yoga class with no music is the stillness, because as you listen to the stillness, mid-way through the class it sounds like rain hitting the floor. Of course the rain is everyone's sweat hitting the mats. Today I heard birds singing outside on the roof, the sweat hitting the mat, and my breath. Life on the mat is wonderful; it has really helped me off the mat with lots of different things. For example, going with the flow, accepting others, accepting myself, accepting the situation and then responding with the right action, it has helped with allowing things, and being present with others. My intuition is stronger, and I find that I am no longer engaged with dramatic people or situations. Also, I seem to be enjoying things as they are. Gossip, judgments, and criticisms of others are a major turn off as well. I can't speak for others; I can only share my experience.

Last night, after teacher Joe's class, a question came up: "Does tomorrow ever really get here?" The answer was that tomorrow will never come, because everything is always happening now. So in practice today, Grant suggested that we knew what pose was coming next, to be honest, I had no idea what was coming next, which speaks volumes. There was a time I was always embracing for the worst, embracing for the next thing to go wrong, looking to play life safe, and why? Because I was concerned by others opinions, getting egg on my face, and wanting to prove I had it together. Life teaches us on the mat, that going with the flow is a lot easier then acting like you have everything under control or even together.

Eyes Closed and a Cup of Joe

Day 84 of 90 straight days of hot yoga at Modo Yoga and I awoke at 4 am and made some coffee, poured my coffee, grabbed my mat and walked my half mile to the studio to practice. I had a wonderful time talking with teacher Joe and others before practice. I then went into the studio, closed my eyes, and teacher Joe invited us to feel the softness of the breath in Child's pose with our eyes closed. I did and could feel the soft breath moving in my body temple. So he asked us to stand up as we started, and I closed my eyes for the entire practice. I noticed with my eyes closed that my standing series was a lot more wobbly, and I also didn't care, because who am I wanting to impress, but I also noticed that with my eyes closed, how the breath is neutral. No judgment. The breath experiences everything and doesn't have time to hold on to anything. With my eyes closed, I had to be present. With my eyes closed there is no more thoughts about how you look, or approval, because you can't see any comparisons outside of you. In fact, at one point I didn't even know I had a body. I just felt energy, and poses became like moving energy. Not like when the eyes are open and it looks like I am moving this body. Also with my eyes open my focus goes to looking at my balance, but with my eyes closed I must feel the balance.

By closing my eyes today I realized why playing it safe, controlling, being neat and tidy with others is important; it is because we are scared of feeling. If I play life safe, then I don't want to feel hurt, happy, alive, or whatever moves through me. Our senses are part of the thinking mind and related to the brain itself. But remove those senses, and you are left to feel and trust. Today, with the eyes closed, I was in the dark, trusting teacher

Joe's voice. And that really enlivened my practice.

I look out in nature, and when I do, I see everything growing at its own pace, and when I close my eyes and practice I can understand why. Life is really meant to be a moment-by-moment experience. The world has another view, which is fine; it is just not one I share anymore. We are all connected. Today I could feel the breath of the entire room breathing. That is powerful.

Groovy

Day 85 of 90 days straight of hot yoga at Modo Yoga LA and I stepped into the studio to take Lisa's class. I love Lisa's style. It is always in the style of the times and she picks the right music as well that fits the class. She reminded us to use the 60 minutes to be present in each pose. So we began.

What I noticed about the importance of being present on the mat and in life is this, by not being present on the mat fully, and in life fully, we tell the universe this is not enough, that we are not enough. We tell the universe that we need more, or maybe there is something missing. We might eat with a friend or be on a date, and we are checking our phones to see if there is something more important than this moment going on. And our dates, friends, and family feel hurt in some way.

I read an article the other day about someone criticizing Eckhart Tolle on teaching "The Power of Now." I realized that we mistake people's passion for being right in the media, in politics, business, and life, yet because people are passionate does not mean they are right. In our day an age, we miss the opportunity to be here now.

If you are at home reading this, sense how your body is, your mind is, right now. Just be aware of how much the mind resists right now. When I am present in the pose and breathing, life is a gift. I give my gift away every time I choose to leave now and worry about something – worry about tomorrow, yesterday, and yet right now there is a gift wanting to be opened, and it is called the present. Give yourself a gift. Be present with everything and everyone today. Watch miracles unfold.

Day 86 of 90

Four to Go

Day 86 of 90 straight days of hot yoga at Modo Yoga and I am excited as I move closer to 90. Frankly when I finished day 30 of 30 I never imagined going for 90 straight days. But here I am, four days away. Today's class was with teacher Grant. When I first started this journey on the mat, my mind would anticipate what was coming, by planning for it. Now I accept each pose as it is, and really have no idea where it is taking me. This practice isn't so much about perfection, control, as it is about breathing and allowing what comes up, to come up and go. I have recognized how hard that can be. One of the things that they tell you upon entering the hot room is to take breaks, and stay in the room. Most of us are not used to taking breaks because that would mean we would have to stop doing and start being with ourselves. So we push through, breathe through, will ourselves to exhaustion, just to prove that we are strong and can do it. But what I have noticed the longer I practice, is that none of that is strength, it is simply being scared, running scared, and not looking into the matter on the mat. Why do we care so much about how we look to others? Why do we control people? Why do we participate in jobs we hate, or dislike? Or even worse, why do we believe that running over people, doing whatever we can to get to the top, cheating and manipulating people just to be famous, is okay?

On the mat we learn that the best way to care for this planet is to care for ourselves from the inside out. Modo is way of being in the world. So how you are on your mat is frankly how you are in life. That may be hard to read, but sit with it. Better yet, sit with yourself in a twist and see how quickly you get agitated because you have to breathe with it. Yoga is not about doing; it is a way of being in the world. It is the Yin and Yang, the heaven and the earth of life.

Day 87 of 90

FYW?

Day 87 of 90 straight days of hot yoga at Modo Yoga LA and I entered the studio with three days to go. Out here in Los Angeles the weather has been hot, and so before entering practice today I had a huge bottle of electrolyte water, and plain water. Staying hydrated is most important for everyone. I tell my under eight-year-old girls before soccer to hydrate, hydrate, and hydrate. Grant led today's practice.

Grant led us through a 75-minute flow practice and it was great. I found myself laughing out loud and smiling more; not taking life too serious, and allowing the practice to happen. Grant was wonderful in reminding us of the power of our breath, and taking our time in the practice. He also invited us to feel our way through, or what my mind translated as "FYW" – feel your way. So when I felt my way through today, I lightened the load and smiled more. When I find myself thinking though, the load is heavy and not so fun. So this was a wonderful reminder to FYW through the practice.

As I move closer to day 90 I have recognized how much more fit I am: I don't tire out as easily, stay clear minded in my practice, my breath is strong, my poses have inner strength, and I am proud of my courage. I am seeing that life is a coming and going. That on the mat is the discovery of now. Yes, there are times when the old pattern wants to come in, but I am aware of it, and allow it to pass.

Modo yoga is a wonderful reminder that life is happening. Right now as you read this, life is happening, meaning the breath is breathing you, the blood is moving through your veins, organs working, heart pounding, lungs taking air in, and yet we don't have to do a thing; those things are just happening now without you. Really, the only thing we have to turn from master to servant is the mind. That is cool! So yoga gives you the opportunity to deal with your mind and as you watch it on the mat, you begin to move closer to who you are. Love it! Love you too!

Day 88 of 90

No Thinking Involved

Day 88 of 90 straight days of hot yoga at Modo Yoga and I entered the studio for a Yin practice with teacher Joe, gearing up for Tuesday's flow with Joe at noon, which is day 90. This morning I spoke at Unity Burbank about my 90-day challenge. Most people would like to know what would happen next, and I am really appreciating the well wishes, emails, and comments as I move towards Tuesday. What I appreciate about this journey is all of you are in on it with me. This is really a community experience.

At Unity today I was surprised by having another yogi there watching my talk, Sid. I talked about acceptance in yoga – unconditional acceptance of where you are, fully engaged in your breath. Your breath is amazing. That is why I feel there is that saying, "You take my breath away." There is no thinking involved on the mat. That might be a good slogan, "Welcome to your yoga mat, no thinking involved, just feel."

Joe brought us through a series of poses for longer periods of time, and reminded us simply of the breath and being here. There is no place to go but here. During these 88 days of falling into the breath, I realize that each day is given to us as a gift, which means we are born to feel, not think. Thinking keeps us from feeling and feeling is about being. We are born to feel, feel everything, but if we feel, we feel we will be weak; but to me, weakness is not feeling, weakness is thinking. Thinking is the servant of the heart, not the master of it.

The breath is the Divine keeping us alive and well.

The Little Things

Day 89 of 90 straight days of hot yoga at Modo Yoga and I entered Matt's flow class. Today Matt set the intention to focus on the little things in practice, for they add up to the bigger picture, which is a wonderful reminder.

Today in flow I was aware of those little things I may be doing in practice, the little foundational things that help out the bigger picture in the practice. I recognized in my practice the importance of different rotations in different poses and since our focus was on twists, I really became aware of the breath. Life is really very simple on the yoga mat, but at first it seems complex. Simplify, simplify, simplify. Simply stay with the breath. The breath will take you where you need to go in life and on the mat. I know it seems so simple, but breathe.

Matt reminded us of the alignment in several poses, which was great. Yes after day 89 I am still growing and learning. It feels as if it will continue that way. My hope is that it does. I always enjoy watching teachers practice with us when they aren't teaching. Sometimes you can catch a glimpse of their postures and learn by watching them.

If I am to be sincere with you and open, I must admit to be one day away from 90 blows me away. This 90-day challenge has been incredible. Most people are still curious of what will happen when it is over, not sure. But let me enjoy the 90th day and I will let you know. This is a celebration for me, not something I should run past to the next thing.

I shared this yesterday at Unity Burbank. When I talked, there were many people who harked on the presence, or being here, and who asked what that felt like. Being is feeling and we are called to feel with life, not think it. Thinking takes you out of the biggest ally you have, your feelings. Sometimes I feel that is why people think too much and worry, because they are afraid to feel how they feel now. Without listening to your feelings, you lose touch with the presence and worry. Your feelings matter! When we feel in yoga practice, we can adjust, because breathing and feeling are tools of the trade on the mat. Because when we are breathing and feeling presently, we accept. The quicker you can accept life as it is, the easier it is to adjust. In yoga we are called to "unconditionally accept" the pose, life, the breath, resistance, right as it is unfolding now.

Ninety and the Invitation

Day 90 of 90 days straight of hot yoga at Modo Yoga LA and I am honored that today's class was with teacher Joe and the Modo flow. Matt, Lisa, Carolina, and Grant showed up to the class and practiced to honor me. They are wonderful teachers at the studio whom I admire. Thank you to Emily B who sent me encouragement but who couldn't make it, because it conflicted with her teaching. I am taking a deep breath now, as my body, mind, and soul collect themselves. It feels like that moment in Breakfast Club when they ask the nerd to sum it all up in a letter.

This journey has been filled with babysitters, scheduling, soccer, life, traffic, work, and so much more. Every day I sat with putting yoga first and figuring out how I could fit practice in. I did that for 90 straight days. This single dad made it work. Every day I shared with you; I offered you my story and reflections of my practice, and what I learned. I am honored you stopped by to read it. And for most of you, it inspired you.

Emily M was my behind the scene angel. There are two moments in my life that I will always take to heart, the first is her encouraging me on day 24: "David go for 90 and see where it takes you inwardly, see what unfolds in you, with your journey." And the second moment was somewhere around day 60 when she was teaching and she came up to me in power pose and whispered, "David what day are you on, 80, 75, you are much stronger than you think, go deeper, have your thighs parallel to the mat." My body was not feeling it, but I did, and because she was cheering me on, from that moment on my practice just got stronger and stronger. So thank you to all the angels who encouraged me.

Teacher Joe, in class today, offered us so much wisdom, and

the practice was wonderful and filled with lots of humor. When I started at Modo three months ago, teacher Joe was telling us about the breath, and today was no different. What I got in practice today was that you breathe, and the only thing that changes is the poses. And as Joe explained today, "The poses come and go, and the breath continues." So it felt wonderful to open up to unconditional acceptance on the mat. The invitation on the mat is always in accepting, allowing, and breathing.

Each pose offers us an experience, and the experience is just that, an experience. These 90 days have given me the opportunity to learn how to accept things as they are. In a society of distractions, in a mind that works on distractions, can I come to practice with the willingness to accept what is? Yoga is about realizing our oneness and that place is here. There is nothing to seek, search for, and look for, because it is all here on the mat. Your mat offers you enough. You can handle it and that is why it is happening.

On my journey, like yours, I ran into many days where everything was off, or on, but it passed, and what I realized is that everything on the mat is passing, it is constant change, like a river, but there is a part that wants desperately to hold on, and that is futile. There is nothing to hold on to. Nothing. And so I would rest in the breath and move on to the next offering on my mat, which is the next pose. Every pose is enough as it is, the breath is enough as it is, this is enough as it is, and you are enough as you are.

Thank you to all the staff and teachers at Modo and Mosksha Yoga. I am honored. Thanks also to the wonderful people at Clover. As tears come down my face, I cannot believe I did this, a breath and a smile. My heart is smiling now. Words cannot express.

I love my talks before class with teacher Joe as we always talk about his garden, which reminds me of life.

To Be Continued...

After the 90 straight days of hot yoga ended, I continued for another 10 days, finishing up my journey at 100 straight days of hot yoga. My first day off yoga, I slept for 12 hours.

What a journey! What a blessing! What a life!

Some people have asked me through emails, "David, why hot yoga?" In my case it wasn't so much of looking for hot yoga, but hot yoga finding me. As I mentioned early in the book, the inspiration came and there it was. Looking back I am so glad it was Moksha/Modo Yoga. I had practiced yoga before I stopped for over 12 years and stopped when the divorce came. I had practiced many styles, and I feel with the style of Moksha/Modo that doing yoga every day, the way it unfolded, is a lot easier in a hot room, rather than a studio where you are working up to getting the body warm. The body opens up quicker in the hot room and it allows you to go deeper.

Also with the style of Moksha/Modo Yoga the emphasis is on the wholeness of the student. I like that. It is never about how you look, or your expression, but arriving into the breath, connecting to the breath, and learning to trust the inner you in guiding your practice.

This journey started out as 30 straight days, then moved to 90 straight days, and it was about my own deepening. Life is continuing as it does and I continue to go to hot yoga. Not every day but about five times a week. In my mind I started "doing" 30 days of hot yoga, and as I suggested in the book I left the "doing" for the practice. Yoga has become a wonderful practice for myself. Life is a practice. So this journey continues. You and I continue.

What I took away from the journey of 90 days was that we have always been right here. That this "monkey mind" wants so badly to be the master of our lives, but we are learning to teach ourselves that it is a servant to the heart. In a world that admires great thinkers, we are moving faster into a world of great people who feel and imagine.

The breath is the "soul" purpose in this book. It is the life of who we are. It heals, takes us deeper, and allows us to see with clarity.

As a dad I love my daughter, she is my light, my love, and brings so much to my days. Our relationship deepened after these 90 days of yoga. Our relationship was good before it started, but now it is just deeper. I give her the space to express, I listen to her fully, and I know she feels safe.

She is seen and heard because I learned how to see and hear myself. I learned how to stand in vulnerability and stay open. And most importantly I learned to appreciate my life and appreciate all life.

Yes the world out there can offer us hopelessness, but there is another way to be, by taking the steps to go inward and discover the inspiration of YOU!

As I finish off this book, I look at a butterfly card my daughter cut out and made me, it says, "Wow Harper, Love you Dad." I wish when we meet each other, we don't say, "Hello" but "Wow! Wow you are amazing!" because you are, each of us is.

Thank you for reading a slice of this life, to be continued...

Acknowledgments

First I want to say thank you to Harper Brown my daughter who taught me and continues to teach me how to love all out with no regrets. You inspire your dad so much and I love you with everything I am.

I would also like to acknowledge the instructors of Modo Yoga Los Angles, for without their love for yoga and heart-centered compassion, this book would have never happened. I thank you Modo Los Angles staff and teachers: Jose, Jess Robertson, Carolina Castro, Emily Buck, Matt Hill, Dalton Grant, Robiwan, Charis Anton, Joe Komar, Deena Robertson, Grant Mattos, Lisa Patino, Angela Granziera, and Emily Morwan for inspiring me to go for 90 days after I did 30. Your love and support on the sidelines was beyond words. Founder Ted Grand thank you for your inspiring words after reading my posts, you walk what you teach and founded.

To O-Books for publishing this book and trusting that people care enough to read it. To those at O-Books who made this possible: Maria Barry, Trevor Greenfield, Stuart Davies, Mary Flatt, Maria Moloney – your eyes and heart in helping me edit this book is such a gift, Catherine Harris, and Dominic C. James.

To my parents Pat and Dave who have stood by my side through thick and thin and kept cheering me on and praying for me. To my sister Kathleen who is always teaching about fierce love, and Charles, Vince, Angelina, and Mariah, you guys rock.

To my Grandma Brown who passed away in March 2014. Thank you for always encouraging me and loving me when everyone I knew walked away during my divorce. Your prayers, inspiration kept me from going to my own death. You saved my life. To the Browns in particular my Uncle Paul who got me to skydive, and my Uncle Steven who showed me the power of prayer when others attack you with words and actions. To the

Telucci family, go giants. Rachel my Godchild I love you. To Uncle Richard, "Who loves ya?"

To John Gloria for his constant support as a friend. To Christina, Candy, Pete, DC Love, Theresa G, Emmanuel Dagher, Anita M, Ophir, Ina, Keith Blanchard, Abigail Noel, Rose, Merry Kain, and the other angels in my life for all their support love and cheerleading. To Nancy O, Rhonda Gola, New Zealand Liz, Yogis everywhere!

To those at Unity Burbank, Christine, Jimmy, Donna, Tommy, Dan, Jim, Bob, and everyone else who celebrated, held, and loved me as I moved through this journey.

To Clover Juice (http://cloverjuice.com/) for supplying me love from the earth, and whose cleanse taught me the importance of eating and drinking organic. You guys rock! A shout to you in Los Angeles on La Brea. To Lulu Lemon who allowed me the opportunity to post on their site my yoga journey and celebrated my 100 days.

To learn more about Moksha/Modo Yoga

MY International Head Office:
Centre for Social Innovation
720 Bathurst Street
Toronto, ON, Canada
M5S 2R4

www.mokshayoga.ca

United States: http://modoyoga.com/

Los Angeles Modo Yoga: http://los-angeles.modoyoga.com/
340 S La Brea Ave, Los Angeles, CA 90036
(323) 938-5000

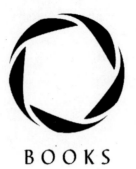

BOOKS

O is a symbol of the world, of oneness and unity. In different cultures it also means the "eye," symbolizing knowledge and insight. We aim to publish books that are accessible, constructive and that challenge accepted opinion, both that of academia and the "moral majority."

Our books are available in all good English language bookstores worldwide. If you don't see the book on the shelves ask the bookstore to order it for you, quoting the ISBN number and title. Alternatively you can order online (all major online retail sites carry our titles) or contact the distributor in the relevant country, listed on the copyright page.

See our website www.o-books.com for a full list of over 500 titles, growing by 100 a year.

And tune in to myspiritradio.com for our book review radio show, hosted by June-Elleni Laine, where you can listen to the authors discussing their books.

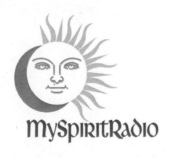

MySpiritRadio